Jo Hemmings was the UK's first Dating Coach and is a Relationship Coach and trained Behavioural Psychologist. She has weekly body language columns in *More!* and *New!* magazines and writes regularly for the national press. Jo makes regular appearances as the sex expert on ITV's *This Morning* and as a celebrity psychologist on BBC and Sky news, and she was the behavioural psychologist on Big Brother from 2008 to 2010. Her websites include:

www.datingcoaches.co.uk
www.celebritypsychologist.co.uk

Sex Games

Fantasies, role play and toys to spice up your love life

Jo Hemmings

Vermilion
LONDON

1 3 5 7 9 10 8 6 4 2

Published in 2011 by Vermilion, an imprint of Ebury Publishing

Ebury Publishing is a Random House Group company

Copyright © Jo Hemmings 2011

Jo Hemmings has asserted her right to be identified as the author of this
Work in accordance with the Copyright, Designs and Patents Act 1988

The Random House Group Limited Reg. No. 954009

Addresses for companies within the Random House Group can be found at
www.rbooks.co.uk

A CIP catalogue record for this book is available from the British Library

Penguin Random House is committed to a sustainable future for
our business, our readers and our planet. This book is made from
Forest Stewardship Council® certified paper.

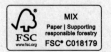

MIX
Paper | Supporting
responsible forestry
FSC® C018179

Printed and bound in Great Britain by Clays Ltd, Elcograf S.p.A.

ISBN 9780091929299

Copies are available at special rates for bulk orders. Contact the sales
development team on 020 7840 8487 for more information.

To buy books by your favourite authors and register for offers, visit
www.rbooks.co.uk

The information in this book has been compiled by way of general guidance
in relation to the specific subjects addressed, but is not a substitute and not to
be relied on for medical, healthcare, pharmaceutical or other professional
advice on specific circumstances and in specific locations. Please consult your
GP before changing, stopping or starting any medical treatment. So far as the
author is aware the information given is correct and up to date as at August
2010. Practice, laws and regulations all change, and the reader should obtain
up to date professional advice on any such issues. The author and publishers
disclaim, as far as the law allows, any liability arising directly or indirectly
from the use, or misuse, of the information contained in this book.

Contents

Introduction

Naughty, kinky, wild, dirty sex. Dressing up, letting your imagination run wild and playing with vibrators, handcuffs and whips. Are fantasies bad, smutty, shameful thoughts that ought to be banished to the darkest recesses of your guilty mind? Do sex toys and games mark you out as some sort of a sexual deviant? Or are they part of a lust-filled, imaginative, fun and joyous sex life shared with someone you trust with your most intimate thoughts and activities?

No prizes for guessing where I stand on this one. Being able to share your deepest desires with your partner should be liberating and exciting, not embarrassing, or viewed as disgusting or abnormal. Whatever goes on privately between two consenting adults should be considered normal. You may not want to do everything your partner suggests – or vice versa – but openness, honesty and being sexually adventurous is key to a passionate, fulfilling sex life, especially in a long-term relationship.

And yet in order to have fun we have to know how to start. Or indeed, how to progress. What will work for us? What will our partner accept and enjoy and what might they find offensive or shocking? How much is too much? And just what is the point of bringing games, props, fantasies and toys into our sex lives?

Sex Games takes you on a gentle yet exhilarating journey to help enhance your sex life through games, fantasies, role play and toys, all accompanied by the sheer power of your imagination. I don't expect you to go from zero to top speed, sexually speaking, in just a few days or even weeks. Or to open up your sexual toy box each and every time you make love. Always remember that spicing up your sex life is not a competition and we all have our boundaries, so make it clear when you've reached your risk, pain or danger limits, or simply reached your own pleasure boundary. *Sex Games* does exactly what it says on the tin: it's about tempting your lust life with fun, pleasure and excitement. But more than that, it's harnessing that zest with some serious (and not-so-serious) know-how, enabling you to empower yourself by managing your fantasies, applying a little role play, appreciating the joy of a sex game or two and understanding how to get the most out of the myriad sex toys out there.

Every game, toy and suggestion in this book has been

tried and tested either by me or my willing team of researchers and everything comes with my personal recommendation. You won't want to try it all – and there may be things that you definitely won't want to consider. You may enjoy the psychological analysis of some of the fantasies mentioned or you may simply want to know which vibrator represents the best value for money. But if just some of the ideas and suggestions contained in the book excite you, whet your appetite, open your mind and manage to banish one of the major causes of relationship break-up – that of a complacent, mundane and predictable sex life – into non-existence then I hope you'll find it all worthwhile.

1 Fantasies

What's the Difference Between Fantasy and Role Play?

Let's start by looking at the fundamental differences between sexual fantasies and sexual role play. If you look up these words on the net – or read basic books about them – you'll find that not only are fantasies and role play used as interchangeable terms, but that sex 'games' get included too!

In truth, fantasies and role play, sexually speaking, are very close to each other. A fantasy is mainly a conscious awareness, sometimes with subconscious roots, a daydream in other words, of something that arouses and excites you. Fantasies are generally private thoughts, and often induce confusion, shame or guilt by the very fact that although we find them sexually arousing, we would never, ever want them to be anything else but 'theatre of the mind'.

Role play, as we'll see in the next section of this book, certainly involves an element of fantasy, but it's something that we do both fully consciously and deliberately, with the agreement, trust and participation of our partner.

FANTASY VS ROLE PLAY

To illustrate these core but sometimes overlapping concepts, these are typical of the standard definitions of fantasy and role play:

Fantasy: Mental images or imaginary narratives that distort or entirely depart from reality. Primary fantasies arise spontaneously from the unconscious while secondary fantasies are consciously summoned and pursued. In adult life it is crucial to creative thinking and the making of art. Fantasy can become destructive if it serves as a constant refuge from the real world and a source of delusions.

Role play: Simulation exercise where the participants act out specified roles in a dramatisation of an event or situation. The purpose of role playing is to achieve better understanding of a situation by experiencing a realistic simulation.

So in the simplest of terms, fantasy is imaginative and unrealistic while role play is practical and realistic.

This chapter will look at the top ten fantasies for men and women, as well as other, more complex – and sometimes worrying to the individual that is having them – fantasies that are also among the most commonly reported. Many of these are reassuringly harmless while others have roots in our childhood and adolescence, which when explained and understood can make individuals feel a lot less guilty or 'abnormal' about having these fantasies.

How Do Fantasies Affect Your Sex Life?

There's a lot written about sexual fantasies – and there are two main schools of thought. One is that having fantasies and sharing these with your partner is a healthy, productive and totally normal part of a fulfilling and varied sex life. However, some believe that simply having fantasies is unhealthy, unpleasant and detrimental to a sex life that takes place in the real world. And that's *before* you choose to share these imaginings with your partner!

I definitely fall into the school of thought that believes having such fantasies is not only healthy, imaginative and fun but it is a vital part of keeping a relationship alive sexually. However, I do have reservations: there are some fantasies that are best kept to yourself for fear of offending or distressing your partner (and you will need to judge this, depending on your lover's views) and/or others that need to remain as fantasies as actually carrying them out could very well be seriously damaging to your relationship. And, of course, there are a few people out there whose sexual fantasies become so disturbing and recurrent, or who feel the need to act out these feelings in an unpredictable and psychotic way, that they must seek psychosexual counselling of some sort.

But in essence, this book considers that the 'normal' range of sexual fantasy and being able to share your deepest desires with your partner should be liberating and exciting. You may not want to do everything your partner suggests – or vice versa – but openness, honesty and being sexually adventurous is key to a passionate, fulfilling sex life, especially in a long-term relationship. Remember: whatever goes on privately between two consenting adults should be considered normal, not embarrassing or disgusting.

So what holds us back from trying something new and different? Basically it's down to fear. Fear of our bodies, of losing control, looking ridiculous or being intimidated by the sheer rawness of this level of intimacy.

Prepare to Share?

We grow up playing as children, but gradually all our games become serious and there's very little playtime left in our adult lives. For some people, fantasies are great mental sex toys, interactive playgrounds for the libido. By allowing yourself your fantasies, rather than trying to suppress them, you will become more in tune with the sort of things that turn you on, which can lead to an enhanced and more imaginative sex life.

So it's important to make friends with your fantasies. Don't vainly attempt to control them, and maybe they won't take control of you. Use them as safe outlets for dark, naughty or forbidden desires that you can't, or wouldn't, want to live out – perhaps because you know that doing so would hurt you or someone you love.

What about sharing? Opening up about otherwise secret sexual fantasies with your partner can make lovemaking more exciting. Sharing fantasies isn't usually necessary when you first have sex together. So much is new in reality, your mind doesn't have to go much further than the present moment for stimulation. But after a while, when you're in a long-term relationship, you get to know each other's bodies so well that your mind is bound to drift into fantasy. After all, there are only so many physical positions into which you can bend your bodies, but there is an endless array of stimulating mind games you can play. On the other hand, as I have said, your secret sexual fantasy could hurt, anger, scare or disgust your lover. One person's fantasy is another person's nightmare.

So sharing really depends on you, your partner and the fantasy. Proceeding with caution is advisable – make playful suggestions and hints rather than spelling out exactly what you want to do. Coming on too strong about your fantasy can seem overwhelming to your partner, make them feel inadequate or even make them feel that they don't really know you at all if you could have been harbouring such a private and 'outrageous' fantasy for such a long period of time.

If you've never shared a fantasy with your lover, and you'd like to try, start by sharing a memory, a thrilling erotic experience that you actually had together. Reminisce about it in bed, and then embellish the memory by imagining something that could have made the experience even more exciting. You can also stimulate the sharing of fantasies by reading or looking at erotic fiction and non-fiction together. You can be explicit, romantic, outrageous and honest, but you must be sensitive to the reactions of your partner. If you can sense arousal and interest from your lover, keep embellishing the fantasy. If you are feeling negative reactions or a physical and emotional withdrawal from your partner, either leave it for another time or step down a gear or two in your expectations of your fantasy world.

Unless you and your lover are fortunate enough to have that rare sort of intimacy – a sublime knowledge of how each other thinks and complete trust in one another's reactions – revealing your fantasies to your partner can be a risky business. But it's a no-pain, no-gain world and it could be a chance worth taking, as sharing your sexual fantasies, with all its myriad possibilities for adventure and fun, can be hugely rewarding in your relationship and the perfect antidote to that curse of so many long-term relationships: regular but predictable or mundane sex.

Is Turning Fantasy into Reality a Good Idea?

The two questions that I get asked most frequently regarding sexual fantasies are: 'Is it okay to fantasise *during* sex?' and 'What happens when a fantasy develops into the real thing?' The first answer is 'absolutely yes', and you'll discover why as you read further.

The second question, however, is a tough call. It is often one partner, more than the other, who drives a fantasy to become a reality and this can cause a serious imbalance in a relationship, especially if there is pressure to turn an innocent-enough fantasy designed to fuel sexual desire and fun into reality. It's also important to remember that there are absolutely no boundaries in the fantasy world, so the reality can be disappointing at best and, at worst, be a fatal blow to a relationship or permanently damage you or your partner's self-esteem. Much of the fallout of your special daydreams becoming reality is down to the fantasy itself. Wanting – and having – an erotic massage is quite different to fancying – and then arranging – a threesome, for example. The success of 'doing it for real' depends on you and your lover's confidence to explore fantasies further as a couple, the strength and durability of your relationship and the ability to deal with any unforeseen consequences in an honest and straightforward way. Which is a very long way of saying that the more complex fantasies should be appreciated for simply being that: a fantasy, a daydream and a tool to stimulate you physically and emotionally during sex. Turning a fantasy into reality won't work unless you and your partner are both of exactly the same mind, with no pressure from one or the other, and are able to weigh up the potential emotional fallout in a mature and open way and accept that it undoubtedly *will* have some effect on your relationship, albeit not necessarily a disastrous one.

The Psychology of Sexual Fantasies

Of all the aspects of human sexuality, the realm of fantasy remains the most elusive. We can feel guilty, confused, shocked and appalled by the power of our erotic imagination. Many of us would feel far more embarrassed admitting to an intimate fantasy than discussing how often we have sex and with whom. We tend to feel less embarrassed about admitting that we might have problems having an orgasm or that we don't really like certain sexual positions. This is partly because we're unsure of what our fantasies say about us. Do they reflect unconscious desires and secret appetites that we'd rather keep private?

And what does it mean if we don't fantasise at all? Or if our fantasies are straightforward and unadventurous? Could it mean that we are frigid or just plain unimaginative? In these supposedly permissive times, there's a lurking suspicion that we should be entertaining all manner of wild and exotic fantasies, and if that's not too exhausting, we should probably be acting them out with our partner, too. Either way, it's a bit of a minefield, and one that probably lies beyond our conscious control.

Statistically, around 96% of British men and 90% of British women report having sexual fantasies, so it may surprise you to know that almost everyone has sexual fantasies, even if they think they don't, as some people dismiss them instantly, rather than allowing them to dwell in their conscious mind. In fact, most of us release our sexual fantasies through our subconscious in the form of dreams. Depending on which school of dream analysis you choose to consider, many seemingly 'innocent' dreams actually represent our sexual selves in one shape or form. Sexual fantasies are a fundamental element of human nature, a primal instinct to imagine and speculate. Some of these erotic imaginings have clear links with what is – or maybe isn't – going on in our sex lives, but many aren't that obvious.

Your 'signature' fantasy

Like a recurrent dream, we often have a 'signature' fantasy, returning – only this time in our conscious, rather than the subconscious state of dreaming – to the same type of fantasy over and over again. We often become conditioned, or comforted, by a similar fantasy repeating itself – whether it's sex with a stranger or being dominated. This is because we end up responding to certain psychological cues and the fantasy sets off our arousal system. This fantasy gets reinforced through orgasm and so we can become attached to a particular scenario associated with pleasure.

This signature fantasy is often related to our earliest sexual awakenings as a young teenager. It has its basis in the longing and yearning of our most formative years, sexually speaking, and comes out in adulthood as sexual fantasy, both in the conscious and in the subconscious.

Like other forms of fantasy, unless it threatens to get out of control or you have ever stronger feelings that the very recurrence is driving you to act it out in reality, embrace and enjoy your recurrent fantasies. Think of them as a draft of a short story – by reviewing and refining them over time, they can become better and better.

Why do we fantasise?

We don't know exactly why we fantasise or indeed how or why they develop. Evolutionary psychologists have suggested that sexual fantasies contribute to sexual arousal, which in turn facilitates procreation. Thus sexual fantasies may play an important, previously unrecognised, role in the continued propagation of the human species. Freudian psychotherapists and psycho-analysts, by contrast, have speculated that our fantasies may have developed as a means both of gratifying wishes and of conquering intrusive memories of early traumatic experiences.

The psychological roots of many of our fantasies begin in the cradle, perhaps even in the womb. By the time you reach your teens, they can become quite intense. Many of your erotic fantasies stem from early memories, the first images that you found arousing. If for no other reason than constant proximity, these images often come through visual or physical interactions with family – your mother's lingerie hanging on the clothesline, your father spanking you, catching your sister naked in the bathroom or your brother wrestling you to the ground. That's one reason why incest fantasies of all kinds are so common. But don't worry – having incest fantasies doesn't mean you've ever really had incest or ever will. While it isn't the place of this book to look in any detail at the psychosexual theories of psychoanalysts such as Freud or Jung, Freud did have a point when talking about the Oedipus and Electra complexes, believing that a lot of our fantasies and development grow from our relationships with our mother or father. The analysis of fantasies – and the related world of dreams – has been part of 'talking therapies' for a long time. Freud also succinctly observed that when two people make love, there are actually four people present: the two people doing it and the two people that they are thinking about!

Your family is not the only source of secret sexual fantasy. You might pick up sensory, almost subliminal, messages from friends, neighbours and school experiences, as well as from your favourite fairy stories, films, adverts, TV shows and music. These early images and messages can be very powerful, because they *occur* when you're at your most formative and impressionable. They become blueprints for your desire, repeating themselves in your memories and activating your imagination, infusing your natural sexuality with meaning and excitement. They alternately confuse, excite, please, comfort and torment you. And they become secret sexual fantasies.

But erotic fantasies can also be influenced by aspects of your early years that weren't so obviously sexual. For instance, if you – or a sibling – were poorly as a child and confined to bed for some significant period of time, you might go on to fantasise about bondage or sensory deprivation. If you were abused or bullied when you were small, then later in life you might turn being bullied into something pleasurable and fantasise about erotic submission or humiliation. On the other hand, your fantasy mind might rather turn the tables on reality and eroticise domination. Your sexual fantasies are keys that unlock the doors of your repressed personal history and in this way are healthy, fun and one of the most positive ways of dealing with past trauma. Like the subconscious world of our dreams, allowing us to let go of some of life's day-to-day anxieties while we sleep, sexual fantasies can offer the same coping strategies – but they allow us to do this in our conscious, waking world.

Are fantasies good for us?

Your fantasies are always with you, playing hide-and-seek with your perceived realities, whispering wild ideas into your inner ear, stirring your passions mysteriously and powerfully. They give you freedom, irrespective of the constraints of the rest of your life: relationships, education, work, family or religion.

Given that most fantasies tend to perfect reality and gloss over our perceived imperfections, one of the primary reasons that we fantasise is to make us appear more sexually attractive and to seem more wanted and desired. This in turn helps us feel more aroused. Sexual fantasies are effective by helping us focus and so enabling us to find sex more enjoyable. In this way, they perform a key role above and beyond the pleasure that they promise. They can help improve our libido, our confidence and enhance our relationships.

If you have a healthy perspective on your fantasies and you manage to achieve fulfilment from them, especially by having an orgasm, they can both act as a release from your current day-to-day stress and anxiety and help resolve traumas from your past. They are also a major benefit in assisting you to relive good sexual memories in a positive, healthy and pleasurable way.

Another encouraging sign that fantasies are good for you is that they are an excellent way of rehearsing or practising for the future. Often known as 'theatre of the mind', these fantasies can encourage and empower you to make the most of sexual adventures that you haven't yet experienced.

For some people fantasies are a way of life and provide pleasure and comfort. For others, it is a more painful experience involving guilt and pain or perhaps coming to terms with a childhood trauma. If your fantasies tend to regularly involve some form of sadism and pain, it may well be that you are dealing with a childhood trauma of some sort, but not necessarily one that was physically abusive. However, dealing with this sort of trauma via a sexual fantasy is of course a far healthier way of processing the experience than those who sadly find that they are unable to contain these thoughts solely to their imaginations and are driven to act on or act out these thoughts, often with tragic consequences.

Understandably, people often would like to get rid of

troublesome fantasies. Maybe they fantasise about playing a submissive, reactive role during sex when really they would like to be more proactive and dominant. Or they might be fantasising about sex with their best friend's partner when they really want to be fantasising about Brad Pitt or their own partner. Trying to banish a fantasy from your mind because it doesn't really suit you can be a difficult process. It is very similar in this respect to our dreams: the harder you try to get rid of an undesirable fantasy from your mind, the more it seems to insidiously return, working its way into your mind and arousing you each and every time your thoughts return to sex. It's a tough thing to control but trying not to worry about it and letting yourself go with the flow is often the quickest way to allowing the fantasy to fade over time and kicking the habit!

Real time or dream time?

But where does fantasy end and reality begin? The philosopher John Richter said, 'Fantasy rules over two-thirds of the universe, the past and the future, while reality is confined to the present.'

Fantasy makes up a huge portion of human consciousness. Memory, as it filters through the mind's eye, is a kind of fantasy that gazes backward, into the past. Hope, anticipation, fear and ambition are fantasies that look towards the future. Our sexuality is fuelled by fantasies of the past and the future, as well as 'pure' fantasies – wild dreams that never happened and that you never really want to have happen – that curiously both haunt and stimulate you at the same time.

There are some fantasies that are really simple desires – the things that you'd like to do with your partner that aren't too 'outrageous' and, once you've taken the first steps to sharing them, will probably become a pleasurable reality for you. And there are others that, if given airtime in the real world, could rock your relationship to the core. A sexual fantasy can be a long, complicated story, a quick mental flash of erotic imagery or something in between. Whatever form it takes, it arouses your sexual feelings and is like the erogenous zone of the mind.

And as I have mentioned on pp. 9–11, while some fantasies are best left as the febrile workings of your mind, others are worth sharing or carrying into the real world. It all depends on the type of fantasy and you and your partner's attitudes towards it.

What Kind of Fantasies Do You Have?

Essentially, most fantasies fall into three broad categories. The first is the daydreaming, 'if only', wishful thinking-type fantasy that might involve you having sex with a celebrity or with someone else that you find attractive, but who is unavailable in some way or for some reason.

The other two most common forms of sexual fantasy work on the principles of sadism or masochism: sadism is the act of deriving sexual pleasure from being dominant and forceful to others, while masochism is quite the opposite and involves being bound, beaten or humiliated in some way to get sexual pleasure. Sadists will have dominant fantasies while masochists will have passive fantasies. A huge amount has been written on how healthy or otherwise these two types of fantasy are, and whether one is 'better' than the other. Clearly it is crucial to have a sense of perspective about sexual fantasies. The mind is a natural place to work through those private desires that the vast majority of us would never consider acting out in real life. It is *only* when the lines get blurred between fantasy and reality, or when the desire to act out violent or subversive fantasies moves into the active, determined part of our brain that problems can occur. If you at any point have fantasies that you sense are beginning to control you – rather than the other way around – it is essential that you visit your GP or a specialised psychosexual counsellor or therapist to discuss these feelings.

Using your imagination

The brain, as you will have gathered by now, is a pretty amazing organ when it comes to having great sex. Without the emotional response, all those nerve endings, all over our skin, when touched, would simply feel like, er, touch. And not very sexy touch at that – more like a doctor checking a reflex reaction than a delicious lover awakening you into arousal. Whether you're with a partner or single, a virgin or an experienced lover, there can be no one out there who hasn't had some tingling of arousal by letting their mind wander to a sexual fantasy, perhaps triggered by something you're reading in a book or magazine, an advert, watching a movie or TV or the simple pleasure of a cool breeze on a summer's day.

There should be no guilt in having these fantasies. If you're single, your imagination is your sexual playground. And if you're in a relationship, you can feel that lustful, naughty edge that fantasy gives you. As I've mentioned, most – but not all – fantasies are best left in your head. They are forbidden pleasures in the main, especially the more explicit ones, with no rules. But although you might feel that some of them are 'inappropriate' – sleeping with a person of the same sex or wanting to be taken by force – these are healthy fantasies that allow our imagination to roam freely and be curious about the world around us. They do not mean literally that we want a homosexual affair or to be raped. Pinning down your assistant over the boardroom table and spreading her legs wide before announcing that you're going to give her the time of her life is a sexy moment of distraction during a mundane working day. In reality you know that you'll be frog-marched out of the building, out of your job and probably in court for sexual harassment in swift order. In fact, sex therapists are generally agreed that providing you can clearly distinguish between fantasy and reality and fully acknowledge the real-time consequences of real-time actions, sexual fantasies are a brilliant and indulgent way of letting off steam without recourse to anything actually immoral or illegal.

Many of us start having sexually based fantasies in our childhood, though we don't really recognise them as being sexual in those pre-pubescent years. I didn't even know what sex really was when I wanted the pop star David Cassidy to take me in his arms and consume me in some way. I didn't want to marry him – I just wanted him, all of him. I was pre-teens, and this gorgeous, floppy-haired boy was my secret longing. The closest I got, of course, was wearing out the paper lips of my poster boy on my bedroom wall as I kissed his image before I went to bed! Then, when I moved on to some other pin-up pop star, David was torn down and replaced by my new desire. And so it is with most of us. Our fantasies evolve in time – one minute we can't wait to deflower a cute-looking schoolboy, the next minute we're after a sexy older guy to impart a little sexual wisdom. And the truth is most of us fantasise about things that we'd hate to happen in reality – would you really want to watch the pizza delivery boy making out with your girlfriend? – but it's a perfect antidote to our normal day-to-day lives, heightening our sexual confidence and allowing our libidos to soar. In fact, the more you fantasise, the higher your sex drive probably is. They're free, available anywhere at any time, can be turned on and off at will and banish all real-life intrusions, from wobbly love handles to worrying about paying the mortgage, into another world. What's not to like?

Research shows that around 90% of us fantasise at some point when we're having sex with a partner. And 90% of people fantasise each and every time they masturbate so it's clear that all sexually active people fantasise at some time or another. Which is encouraging news because the same research shows that those people who do regularly fantasise have more fulfilling sex lives than their less imaginative counterparts.

How to get what you want

So, given that all these fantasies are healthy for our sex lives and to be encouraged, and being honest, upfront and communicative with your partner is one of the best ways to a satisfying sex life, is it okay to tell your partner your fantasies? As I've mentioned on pp. 9–11, it's perhaps the one area of our sexual lives where it's definitely best to proceed with caution. Revealing your own personal fantasies can send your sex life through the roof. It can make it sizzle with variety and excitement. But on the other hand, admitting your fantasies can destroy your relationship. If your partner doesn't share your enthusiasm for a particular fantasy, it can make him or her feel inadequate, insecure and jealous. This is where a clear definition between role play and fantasy is necessary (see p. 6). Fantasies are essentially private thoughts; role play is a shared affair, where the two of you can participate together in playing out a particular scenario. Unless you know your partner very well and can accurately gauge their reactions, my advice is to keep fantasies reasonably private. And even more so if it involves someone you actually know. Admitting that you fancy a celebrity, who you are very unlikely to meet, is very different to revealing that you'd like to have sex doggy style, strapped into a gimp suit, with your partner's best friend.

But if you do want to reveal your fantasy, or indeed want to consider acting it out role-play style, then like anything slightly 'delicate' – who's going to whose parents for Christmas dinner, for example – you need to choose your moment wisely. You need to find a moment that's relaxed, private and intimate. Maybe tell your partner that you had an amazing dream last night (okay, small white lie, it is a dream, just a day version) where something incredibly sexy and surprising happened. See if they react positively to that before going any further. Or ask them if they have any special fantasies – but be prepared for an answer that you might not have wanted or anticipated. Take it a step at a time – fantasies are always easier to act out if you both share a common goal. If his fantasy is to have his testicles massaged with baby oil and yours is to be spit roasted by the entire England football team, then it might be better to keep them as private thoughts after all.

Before I look at sexual fantasies in more detail, it's important to remember that, given that this is a book intent on offering up pleasure, opportunity and fun within your relationship, I have neither attempted to cover every possible variant on sexual fantasies nor a deep psychoanalytic insight into the sexual psyche of those that are having them. There are other books out there which offer a more academic or case-study approach to sexual fantasies and as a psychologist and relationship expert I am neither inclined nor qualified to go into this much depth. Also I have not covered what may be considered to be the more problematic or deviant forms of sexual fantasy generally restricted to men, such as the wearing of nappies and being treated like a baby, asphyxiation or incest fantasies.

Dominance and Submission Fantasies

Dominance and submission, or power and surrender, fantasies are quite common among both men and women. They can range from being romantic and passionate to crude, severe, shocking and even dangerous. Dominance and submission may involve bondage, domination, sadism and masochism (BDSM), an imagined abduction, a safe rape fantasy, spanking, whipping, tickling, torture, teasing, body worship and a host of other activities that may or may not entail actual sexual intercourse.

Bondage is a classic male fantasy, only this is usually where you take control and tie up your partner, rather than being tied up yourself. Which is good news, given that most women usually want to be tied up! Bondage fantasies are dreams involving power and control. In the twenty-first century, where some men feel that their alpha male masculinity is under threat, this fantasy has become ever more common. Inflicting pain through whipping and spanking is another part of the bondage fantasy, as it's the ultimate control and relates to the pain–pleasure axis that is never very far apart during S & M sex.

Many role plays, as we'll see in the next chapter, are based on dominance and submission fantasies, whether it's master and French maid, boss and employee, teacher and pupil, doctor and nurse or whatever dramatic variant you might choose to act out with your partner.

Domination

It's easy to understand why people enjoy dominating others. Power is an adrenalin rush, a sexual, high-risk roller coaster of a sensation, especially in sexual fantasy. You get to do whatever you want to the sex object of your dreams. Or they get to arouse you in any way that you wish. What's not to like?! Traditionally, domination is considered a male fantasy, probably most popular among young men who are relatively powerless in real-life society, even though they have testosterone-pumping energy to spare. But more and more women are enjoying dominant fantasies. This can range from the simple act of sitting on top of your lover, riding him, while remaining both in control of the pace of your love-making and of his pleasure, to tying up and gagging your helpless lover, while you spank him with a whip or paddle until he is completely at your mercy. Some women also like using a strap-on dildo, so that they can anally penetrate their man and reach his G-spot, giving him pleasure while maintaining their control and dominance at the same time.

Submission

But what of submission fantasies? What makes a person want to submit to someone else's control, rather than stay in the driving seat themselves? Why do people long to submit? It's a common fantasy of those who are in control in their real lives. They may be high-powered, successful people at work, responsible for managing a large team of people. Or they might be people who have accepted, through necessity or choice, to assume control of their children or other family member's well-being. Fantasising about being dominated is a chance to surrender and allow someone else to assume this power and responsibility. In their erotic imaginations, and sometimes in a real-life role-playing session with a dominatrix, they surrender control for a brief period in their busy, power-packed day or week. It's like taking a holiday from real-life stress and the responsibility of being in charge, or it's a journey back into a former, younger life where they were under someone else's control. In this way, submission fantasies can be a real stress buster. Society puts pressure on us to be high achievers and success is often measured by our place in society or position at work. Most people don't achieve their position of power especially easily – it can be a long hard graft – and perhaps it is not surprising that it comes as a pleasurable relief to surrender to someone else's control and let them take responsibility for a while.

Being tied up or harnessed to a bed or a chair where you have little chance to move and you are completely at the mercy of a man is the secret fantasy of many women. It allows you to be naughty and enjoy teasing, spanking and whipping without being able to do anything about it. If you feel any guilt about the pleasures of S & M in the real world, your out-of-control fantasy will allow you to indulge it, guilt free.

Another major reason as to why submission is such a popular fantasy is that it allows us to give in to our deepest sexual desires, without feeling any guilt. Whether you are being ravished, abducted, bound up, spanked, tortured, forced to dress like a slut or led around on a leash as the slave of a powerful, sexy master or mistress, in a submission fantasy you get to be made to do what you secretly desire.

Watching Porn

Lots of men fantasise about watching porn with their partner and the truth is that they are pleasantly surprised by the reaction – lots of women love watching porn as much as men and find it a real turn-on. But how do you suggest this in the first place and what kind of thing should you watch?

If you're a guy who is used to watching porn to masturbate, you need to take a little care over your first foray into watching porn with your partner. You might be used to seeing the perfectly formed pink hairless vaginas, over-inflated breasts and platinum hair extensions so beloved by the porn industry, but the chances are that your partner might feel a bit insecure the first time she sees them. My feeling is to go for 'natural', fairly soft porn, where the girls look like proper girls and no surgical enhancements are allowed. Or start with a mainstream movie that has some hot sex in it or classic sex films that can be rented at your local DVD store. Or go online and do a little research into what kind of porn you could be buying into. As a rule of thumb, anything directed by a woman is usually a little softer than those movies made by men! This is a progressive fantasy – start gently and move on up to the harder stuff at a pace that suits you both.

Watching porn together can be good fun. It's exciting, it's naughty and it can show you things visually that you might want to have a go at. But some porn is so awful that you may well find yourself giggling nervously and finding it hugely unsexy. And I am always reminded of Erica Jong's comment to *Playboy* magazine in the seventies, on the perils of watching stereotypical porn movies: 'My reaction to porn films is as follows: after the first ten minutes, I want to go home and have sex. After the first twenty minutes, I never want to have sex again for as long as I live.'

One of the important things to remember about watching porn movies is that they are not meant to be watched with a family bucket of popcorn in your lap and your mind on the plotline. They should be there in the background to excite you and your partner while you masturbate together or in turn or take turns to give each other oral sex while your partner watches the film. If you both want to watch the movie together, get in a position that allows you to have sex as well as both watching the TV – doggy style or woman on top, facing away from her lover, both work well.

The harder core porn, or the brief snippets of wham-bam MILF action that you find on many porn sites, may well suit you when you want a snatched opportunity to masturbate, but these are generally not the kind of movies that you want to share with your partner. Try watching a sexy mainstream DVD with an erotic theme like Michael Winterbottom's *Nine Songs*, Ang Lee's *Lust, Caution* or Steven Shainberg's *Secretary*. Or go for the gentler sort of porn directed by women such as Petra Joy's *Sexual Sushi*, *Female Fantasies* and *Feeling It* or Anna Span's *Southwark Sugar*, *Hoxton Honey* and *Toy With Me*. You can even choose the rating of your movie by these talented directors: R18 for full-on action and an 18 certificate if you want something a little tamer!

Making porn

Instead of watching porn with your partner, how about making your own movie instead? Men especially love the idea of starring in their own porn movie. Part of the fun is planning and then acting out the movie on your very own video camera. This is a harmless, natural fantasy – and one that adds a lot of spice to a couple's sex life as they can get an extra turn-on by enjoying watching it afterwards. One word of warning, especially for women: if you are going to make a tape, keep it in a safe place. Or delete it afterwards. Some men love to show the movie to their mates after a few drinks – it's that showing-off thing that makes him look like a hot stud muffin!

There are a number of books available on amateur filmmaking and some specifically for making your own home videos – porn-star style. Or you can use the video application on your phone. The idea is to make something that's fun, adventurous and will spice up your sex life. You're not after a BAFTA award-winning, full-length arthouse movie!

The award-winning erotic film maker Petra Joy (www.petrajoy.com) has written an excellent book *How to Shoot your Lover* (HarperCollins, 2007), now sadly out of print, and these are her top ten tips on how to make a home movie, porn-style (permission granted by author):

1. **Take control of your camera**

   Switching off the auto settings and choosing the manual exposure, focus and white balance on your video camera will enhance the quality of your video footage.

2. **Go for mystery**

   By shooting through material you will find it easier to capture shadows or reflections. In erotica showing less is often more. Start collecting interesting props that help to tell a story.

3. **Dare to change your point of view and vary your shots**

   This keeps your visuals interesting and you will be able to edit your video footage more creatively.

4. **Try to forget . . .**

   . . . about what you know or have seen about stereotypical glamour models and porn stars. See your models with fresh eyes. Encourage them to do what they enjoy rather than trying to turn them into a porn-star clone. 'Deep throat' or 'double penetration' is not everyone's cup of tea!

5. **Direct your models**

   Never assume whoever is playing for you in front of the camera will know instinctively what to do.

It is not enough to just 'point and shoot' if you want to create stylish and sexy images that are more than just your average 'reader's wives' shots. It is a skill to know when to hold back as a director and let the action flow and when to encourage or gently suggest a change of action.

6. **Don't get too hung up ...**

    . . . about the 'hard-on'. If your models are enjoying themselves, they will forget about the camera and an erection will come naturally.

7. **Forget about the 'money shot'**

    To me the idea about great sex is that you lose control and just enjoy yourself, rather than time your orgasm for the camera. Don't compromise the performers' orgasms for a 'cum shot'.

8. **Allow yourself to be inventive, creative and playful**

    Express your vision of erotica rather than copying someone else's ideas. Do the kind of porn that turns you on. It can also be empowering for a woman to take control and get behind the camera.

9. **If you aim to publish your film**

    Get a signed release form and photocopies of passports from all participants. Generally, though, it is best to keep your home movies for personal use only, so to avoid any public showings of your movies on social networking sites – youporn is a favourite of the slighted lover – post break-up, keep your movie in a very safe place.

10. **'The answer to bad porn is not "no porn" but "good porn"' (Annie Sprinkle)**
So if you have not found what you are looking for in erotic films, make your own. Empower yourself by creating rather than consuming.

More Fantasies

The best lover in the world . . .

The most popular sexual fantasies among men and women involve images of sex with a passionate, attractive, exciting partner who will do whatever you want, even if that means dominating you. The best lover in the world will always please you and leave you feeling satisfied and fulfilled. He or she could be someone you know; it could even be your real-life partner. It could be a past lover, a celebrity or someone who you both idolise and idealise from afar. It could be someone that is strictly out of bounds – a friend's partner or even a relative. The main characteristic of 'the best lover in the world' is that you find this person completely irresistible, at least in your fantasy world.

Even if the sweep-you-off-your-feet, debonair doctor in charge is your Mills & Boon-type fantasy, you will still wonder about this amazing lover, this perfect man who can capture passion, romance and power in his every breath. While such a scenario might involve nothing more than a passionate kiss, the fantasies can also entail sexual intercourse in every position imaginable. The best lover gives the most divine oral sex, adores it when you give it to him, both gives and receives hand jobs that take your libido through the roof and is never averse to the pleasures of anal sex. In addition to these basic physical sex acts, there are many other types of sex about which you might fantasise, especially if you feel deprived of a particular favourite activity or desire.

The Mills & Boon fantasy is gentle and traditional. It's the type of escapism found in old-fashioned romantic novels. It's the dishy doctors and heaving bosom combo, often combined with a lot of eye contact, eyelash fluttering and deep sighs. Or it could be a moonlit walk, hand in hand with a delicious, dark, brooding man who only has eyes for us, along a perfect, soft, sandy beach. It's a lovely and romantic form of escapism and one fantasy that many women, understandably, are happy to confess to.

Oral sex

Men generally have major fantasies about being given – rather than giving – oral sex. And in his fantasies, the woman will be doing it because *she* finds it so pleasurable, and not just to give him delight. She will fall upon his penis with relish and unabated desire, gasping with pleasure and showering his manhood with compliments while consuming it with sublime delight and greedily gulping down his semen with the kind of ecstasy it so rightly deserves. Again, this is often fuelled by porn movies where sex is frequently interrupted by the overwhelming desire of the woman to go down on her man midway through sex. Many men also fantasise about holding a woman by her hair, or pushing her down harder, while she gags on his penis, due to the delicious and irresistible enormity of its length and girth!

Sex with your current partner

It's even more common to fantasise about your real-life lover, who may not be the best lover in the world, but is certainly familiar, exciting and easy enough to conjure up in your erotic imagination. Fantasising about what we would like our partner to do to us – or what we would like to do to them – when we next see them or when we're actually having sex with them – keeps our sex lives and libidos fresh and vital. And, of course, one of the lovely aspects of this type of fantasy is that it's all there for the sharing . . .

Sex with a virgin

Fantasising about deflowering a virgin is common for both men and women. It's all about power, dominance and imparting your sexual wisdom to an innocent party so that they can go out into the world and use that wonderful experience to share with other lovers. We also enjoy fantasies about being deflowered. Playing the innocent virgin, shy and coy and longing to be taught the sexual ways of the world, is very appealing, especially if our own first time wasn't quite the romantic scenario of being swept off our feet by a gorgeous, confident lover with the sexual prowess and sensitivity of a Hollywood movie star. Which, let's face it, is a pretty unlikely scenario in the real world.

But this is definitely a fantasy that you can play out with your lover. As a woman, you can be the seducer by wearing a sexy little outfit of pencil skirt, sharp white blouse teasingly undone to your cleavage and killer heels.

You could play any sort of role where you're the dominant partner – a boss interviewing him for a job or perhaps he's a young boy just looking to do a spot of gardening for you. Or you can reverse roles, where you are the sweet innocent, wearing a prim little blouse buttoned to the neck or a schoolgirl outfit, and your partner is your teacher or boss. There's much more on the playing out of fantasies on pp. 101–26.

Sex out of the bedroom

That this even counts as fantasy at all will shock some 'Martini' people who are happy to have sex any time, any place, anywhere . . . But others, even if they are sexually adventurous in bed, with a world of fantasies playing out in their imagination, simply wouldn't contemplate a fantasy that takes place outside of the bedroom. Think about having sex – or any sexual play – while in a lift, in your office, in a restaurant or café toilet or in a changing room. And if the element of risk seems too much, look closer to home for your fantasies. How about sex in the shower, over the dining-room table, on the kitchen work surface or on the sitting-room floor?

Sex outdoors

Having sex outdoors is becoming something of a forgotten pleasure. In previous generations, when we lived with our parents for longer and when pre-marital sex was still an issue, outdoor sex was much more common. Whether it was in the car, in a secluded car park, in a field on a sunny day or on the beach, behind a handy sand dune or two, having sex in the great outdoors was much more commonplace, borne out of necessity. Where else were you going to go for your illicit pleasures?

These days when we have our own homes and it's easy to book a hotel – and the embarrassment and punishment for being caught having sex outdoors might put the fear of God into us – we can treasure it as a perfectly acceptable fantasy. Although of course if it is such a major imaginary turn-on, the pounding hearts, fresh air and the adrenalin rush of being caught out might simply add to the excitement if you decide to play this one out in real time.

Do remember that it's illegal to have sex in public and it can carry a jail sentence if you're caught and reported. So if you choose to make this particular fantasy a reality, you've got to be sensible about it – take simple precautions like covering yourselves with a picnic blanket and keep to a secluded place, well away from families enjoying a picnic or a day on the beach. So if you're clever and discreet, you can indulge yourselves in the thrill and pleasure rush that al fresco sex offers up. Fantasising about outdoor sex covers so many different places and positions, so it's worth looking at those that you might really enjoy in the real world – as well as avoiding some of the potential trouble that reality can bring with it . . .

In the car
Sex in the back seat of a car, in a dark secluded car park, used to be a bit of steamy-windowed fun. Sadly these days it's got itself a bit of a sleazy reputation, thanks to the reports of a few high-profile celebs who have been caught 'dogging' in car parks. Not to be confused with 'doggy style', dogging is the practice of having sex in a semi-public place with a view to being watched, rather than in seclusion and privacy, or simply going along to watch others.

Car parks frequented by the dogging fraternity are often well known, so if you're going for a little back-seat action these car parks are best avoided. Try a quiet street or country lane instead. Sex in a car can be fun – you can't do it missionary style (unless you've got some fancy rear-seat-folding-flat affair in your car) so you have to get into all sorts of athletic and unlikely positions to avoid gear stick, door handle or seat belt related injuries! So it's definitely a challenge . . .

However, it's much sexier to have sex on the car bonnet. Sure, it's much more risky too, being that much more exposed, but that just adds to the thrill. It's sensible to choose a quiet country lane or similar. Make sure that the car engine is cool – if you've been driving around for a while, it could be bottom-searingly hot. And if you're doing it from cold, make sure you put a coat or a blanket over the top, when the reverse can be true on a chilly day!

The bonnet is the perfect height for the woman to jump up and lie or sit down on, with her legs open, while her man stands in front of her. She can pull him into penetrative sex by wrapping her legs tightly around his middle.

On the beach

The thing that makes sex in the sand so erotic and exciting is in part due to the fact that beachside holidays are already imbued with a massive sense of romanticism and escapism, so just the thought of sex in the sand can make your toes tingle. Plus most people are already semi-naked, enjoying the comforting warmth of the sun and taking pleasure in those long, languid lazy days.

Massaging sun lotion into each other is a fabulous way to kick-start sex in the sand, and you can sculpt sand into the kind of dip and shape that makes it most comfortable to have sex. And sex on the beach after a few hours lazing in the sun means that the deliciousness is all the more intense as your sun-warmed bodies entwine with each other. Of course, one of the downsides to having sex on the beach is gritty, coarse sand ending up deep in the crevices of some especially sensitive places, so the finer the sand the better. You can use a blanket or a towel, of course – or even a sun lounger – but if you do find sand creeping into some of your genital folds, simply enjoy the pleasure of showering it off together once you get back to your home or hotel. And you thought Sex on the Beach was just a sickly-tasting cocktail . . .

In the sea

The sea – or a secluded pool – is a fabulous place to enjoy sex. The water disguises anything going on below neck or waist level and we all feel supple and agile in the water, due to the feeling of weightlessness and buoyancy.

You can have sex deep out to sea – after diving from a boat – or in the shallow end of a pool or you can recreate that wonderfully romantic scene from the Hollywood movie *From Here to Eternity* by rolling about in the sandy shallows of the lapping waves, on the shore, feeling the sea on your naked bodies as it pulls back and forth.

In the garden

Most people love the earthy, clean smell of freshly mown grass with its connotations of summer days of promise and expectation. So what better place to throw down a picnic blanket and make love. The fresh air makes us feel energised and happy and we associate playing in the garden with being a child and the freedom that went with that period of our lives.

If you're lucky, you'll have a nice secluded garden with mature shrubs, a lawn and patio area and little chance of curious neighbours overlooking your al fresco activities. If not, then try it after dark or consider that maybe the thought of being seen might just add to the frisson of it all.

You can do anything on the grass that you could do on the carpet and most things that you can do on a bed, so let your imagination take over.

Or use your patio or picnic table as a prop. Place a rug or duvet down on the table, lie or sit down, and the woman can wrap her legs around her man as he stands in front of her.

On a boat

Of course a boat could mean anything from a small fishing or rowing boat up to a multi-storey cruise liner. One thing they all have in common is that seductive, relaxing, bobbing motion of the sea – unless of course you're in a Force 10 gale, in which case the experience could be somewhat different!

Generally boats are sexy, romantic places with a soft breeze on deck and if you're doing it at night there might be a vast star-studded sky to look up on too. There are all those handy props around as well. Safety rails to hang on to and padded deck loungers to take any potential discomfort away. What could be lovelier than having sex on a boat?

On the hotel balcony

Whether you're staying at the smartest of upmarket hotels or a simple country apartment, a balcony usually gives you fabulous views of the surrounding area as well as being secluded enough to not be too high risk at getting caught out.

Take out a bottle of champagne, something lovely to eat like strawberries, chocolate or olives and indulge yourselves as the sun sets. Then either put the duvet or a thick blanket down on the balcony floor – they're usually made of pretty stern stuff like marble or concrete, so protect your sensitive parts – and snuggle under the stars to be as naughty and as daring as the mood takes you.

Sex with a work colleague

However senior you are at work or however busy, I suspect that there isn't one of us who hasn't daydreamed about what a work colleague might be like in bed. We spend a lot of time, in a non-sexual way, with colleagues of the opposite sex – often considerably more time than we spend with our own partner – fuelling all sorts of imaginings during a mundane or dull working day, or during a business meeting, and this fantasy expresses a natural curiosity about parts of their other lives that we don't have access to and what they might look like with their clothes off. Often these fantasies have you playing the dominant role – either showing your boss exactly what you're really capable of outside of the work environment or assuming a senior role, both in and out of the bedroom, to someone that you manage. These fantasies can also have you taking a more passive role – especially if you have a responsible, senior role in your job – where a work colleague assumes all responsibility for giving you pleasure in whichever way they choose.

Sex with a stranger

The fantasy of sex with a stranger means raw, unadulterated sex. Unsullied by the burdens of everyday life and unfettered by the emotional demands of a relationship, this is pure no-strings-attached sex. You can be as naughty as you like and say and do as you please. You can take over the reins or let the stranger have complete control. For many women, it is the complete unfamiliarity of the man involved that drives this fantasy. There's no fear of rejection, no fretting about whether they'll want to see you again or whether you were a disappointment in bed. It allows you to avoid commitment issues and lets you behave in a way that is never going to have any repercussions that you might encounter within a traditional relationship. One of the reasons that these kinds of fantasy lovers are so appealing is that you don't know anything about them at all.

Men especially find something very appealing about having anonymous sex with a stranger. You might fantasise about catching someone's eye in a hotel bar and, without speaking a word, you give her a signal and she follows you up to your hotel bedroom. Or it might be a woman you see on a regular train journey and you let your eyes and mind wander to her breasts and mouth, wondering what she'd be like giving you oral sex. This kind of fantasy totally avoids commitment issues or fears of inadequacy or performance anxiety. It allows you to have a woman as if she were a prostitute, but without the need to pay as she clearly finds you so desirable and sexy that there is no need to sully the occasion by a tawdry exchange of money.

Sex with a celebrity

This was probably one of your earliest fantasies. Along with fancying the boy or girl next door, or the person who sat next to you at school, most of us had the hots for a pop star or a movie star. They are unreal, perfect, always immaculately turned out, powerful and success-ful. A heady brew. Celebrities always seem to lead a charmed life and are inevitably more interesting and exciting than our current decent but not-that-exciting partner. In reality, they probably have the same issues as the rest of us and bear scant resemblance to the person that their PR machine wants us to think that they are. But they're cute, sexy and you're never going to meet them. So they can't judge you either. Fantasise away . . .

Being seduced by an older partner

This is typically and more likely to be a male fantasy. A lot of younger men want a fast track to sexual experience without the commitment of a relationship first. The older woman scenario provides perfect fodder for this fantasy. A woman who has wisdom and a whole, as yet undiscovered by you, repertoire of sexual expertise, is old enough to know what she wants and not be too modest to go for it and who can see that a proper relationship would be out of the question, due to the age gap, is the perfect solution. For some men, this was an early sexual fantasy – often fancying your best mate's mum, a neighbour or a teacher at school – and one that they enjoy returning to.

Sex with someone of the same sex

It's tempting for men to think that women often have this fantasy (it means much more chance of the promise of girl-on-girl action or at least the description of what she'd like to do with another girl) and indeed many women do fantasise about lesbian sex, especially with someone gorgeous. There is something hugely appealing about having sex with someone whose bits are the same as yours and every day we're bombarded with images of lovely women in magazines, on TV and in the movies, so it's natural to be curious. When fantasising about sex with another female, most women imagine the other woman's whole body – her breasts, bottom, mouth, hair, vagina, clitoris, soft skin, seductive eyes, and so on – whereas when men fantasise about other men, they tend to focus solely on one part, their fantasy partner's penis. And unlike a man fancying another man, society is much less 'lesbian phobic' than it is homophobic, which somehow makes it seem a whole lot more acceptable.

Sex with a woman can be immensely pleasurable as it can be a more tender and less urgent experience than sex with a man. Most women also seem to have an easier time accepting their bi-curious fantasies than most men do. Whereas some of this acceptance lies in the fairly recent portrayals of women kissing or fondling on TV soaps and dramas, women know that most men are turned on by two women together, whereas it's still a rare, liberal and open-minded woman who enjoys two men together. Additionally, there are also greater health risks involved in same-sex lovemaking between men, due to the majorly increased chance of penetrative sex.

But it's also natural for men to be bi-curious. It doesn't mean you're gay or homophobic. It's an incredibly common fantasy, for both sexes, during adolescence and the taboo that comes with it (especially for men) is bound to make them remain curious. It's naughty, it's 'wrong' (of course it isn't, but it feels 'wrong' for most heterosexual men) and so it's inevitable that it ends up as a fantasy – which is simply our mind toying with something experimental that arouses us without any feeling of guilt. Like many fantasies we probably won't actually do it – or even want to do it – but it's healthy to be aware of those sexual options that are available to us, should we wish to pursue them.

Sometimes people fantasise about a threesome, all of the same sex, which is simply a more daring and racy version of fantasising about a more intimate, same-sex twosome. Or maybe the third lover is simply there for show, to guide you on what to do with someone of your own sex. The sexperts Masters and Johnson believed that heterosexuals often fantasise about homosexual encounters and vice versa, more often reflecting curiosity and other impulses than the desire to change the gender of one's real-life lovers.

Fantasising about someone of the same sex doesn't mean that you're gay – although of course it could mean that, especially if you might be masking or repressing desires for someone of the same sex. It probably does represent genuine bisexuality but the truth is that almost all of us – whether we embrace it in our imagination or on a more real level – have some element of potential bisexuality within us. The eminent sexologist Alfred Kinsey was among the first to do extensive research on this, and his results revealed that we're all on a bisexual continuum with absolute heterosexuals on one end and absolute homosexuals on the other end. Very few of us fall at one extreme or the other and while most of us are bisexual to some degree, it simply means that we exercise this bisexuality in our imaginations rather than in real life.

Like many other types of fantasy, it is liberating repressed feelings whether these are in your conscious, aware mind or lying dormant in your subconscious. It doesn't mean that you ought to do it either. Same-sex fantasies can signify a lot of different things for people who lead mostly straight real lives – from simple curiosity about how their own bodies work to the desire to break conventional social taboos.

Watching and being watched during sex: voyeurism and exhibitionism

Like being bi-curious, most of us have wondered what it would be like to watch someone else having sex. Sure, we can see sex on the telly any night of the week, but that's acting sex. It's not really happening. It's just for the cameras.

But what if you could watch your best friend and their partner having sex? How do they do it? You might have drifted off into the fantasy of wondering what your partner's best mate was like in bed, so what if you could see what they were really like? Voyeurism fantasies involve being watched while you're having sex or maybe being forced to have sex in front of other people. You might also be the one spying on someone else having sex. Anyone, a stranger or someone you know, can be the subject of this fantasy. You would be ashamed – maybe ruined – if anyone ever found out. But it's the risk element that helps make it feel so good!

Watching another couple have sex, especially when they don't know they are being watched, is both exciting and forbidden. Sex is meant to be private and invading this privacy by spying on someone is high taboo, however much you talk about what you do on girly nights over a bottle or two of wine or down the pub with your pals. It's an absolutely natural, understandable curiosity and provided you don't intend to carry it out by shimmying up the drainpipe to look in your neighbour's bedroom window, Peeping Tom-style, it's a perfectly healthy fantasy.

Another common fantasy is being seen and showing

off while having sex. This is known as exhibitionism. Most exhibitionism and voyeurism is about the joy of the erotic gaze and the thrill of being gazed upon, breaking through the strong social taboo of visual privacy.

The entire porn industry is based on people's voyeuristic desires to see otherwise forbidden images of other people engaged in sex. There are obviously enough people who love to be watched because there are plenty of porn stars and strippers. Those are extreme professions to be in, but in fantasy you can do it all and bare it all before thousands or in forbidden places.

With the advent of reality shows, erotic blogs, easily accessible free porn and obsessive, sexy photo-posting on social-networking communities, exhibitionism and voyeurism are becoming less and less about fantasy or reality and more about media influence, as 'ordinary' people can morph into exhibitionists just by making and posting their own porn, turning everyone on their friend list into voyeurs, if they so choose.

It's commonly believed that exhibitionism is a female fantasy, while voyeurism is male. Understandable, really, when most online pornography as well as pay-per-view porn movies are produced for men's delectation, strip- and lap-dancing clubs have female performers for male customers and the great majority of straight sex magazines and websites have pictures of women for men to admire. The internet is changing this perception, but traditionally women tend to be the ones who get paid for sex as a stripper, prostitute, porn star, mistress or other sexual performer.

Yet in nature, it is the traditional role for the male to be the exhibitionist. Male birds – the peacock for example – have the brightest, most gaudy plumage designed to attract a female during elaborate 'seduction' displays. Whereas women can get away with overtly sexual outfits and virtually every conventional role-play scenario involves the women, rather than the man, dressing provocatively, men get very few – legal, anyway – opportunities to sexually display themselves for women in our society. They want to share just how adept they are at making love, especially if another woman is watching, and of course, being a fantasy, their sexual skills naturally rival that of the hottest porn star on the planet!

So it has become much more common for men to secretly fantasise about exhibitionism. They desperately want to show themselves off, with special emphasis on their taboo penises that are so forbidden everywhere except hardcore porn. This has led rise to a relatively new phenomenon in the fetish world, with many websites devoted to it, known as Clothed Female, Naked Male (CFNM).

Sex with another person other than your partner

This is one of the most common sexual fantasies of all, especially if you've had few partners in your life or have been with someone a long time. This could be a stranger, a celebrity, a friend or more often than not a past lover. If you look back in your life, you might find that however much you love your current partner or however fabulous he or she is in bed, the actual sex that you had with someone else was technically better. This is reassuring and normal. Psychologically, we tend to go for a long-term partner that has a number of attributes that we're looking for, whether that's kindness and consideration, reliability and honesty, intelligence or sense of humour. If he or she also happens to be the hottest partner that you have ever had sex with then you have truly hit the jackpot – most of us tend to accept the sex is wonderful, but not necessarily the best ever.

Sometimes fantasising about having sex with another partner is simply daydreaming about what that person would be like in bed. If it's a former lover, we tend to reignite memories of how great the sex with them was. As a fantasy we allow ourselves the privilege of filtering those memories, so that we don't dwell on all the bad times we might have had with that partner; we simply concentrate on how good the sex was. This 'rose-coloured glasses' form of fantasy is to be encouraged as it stops us mourning the loss of a past lover, but releases negative thoughts by allowing ourselves to reminisce about the good times in our minds.

It's also one of the most common and most simple male sex fantasies. It's the grass is greener on the other side scenario, only you can indulge in it without any consequences or fallout from your current partner. You might fantasise about a woman with huge breasts, a forbidden woman like your partner's sister or a prostitute or even a virgin that you can seduce and teach all things sexual to last them a lifetime . . .

Playing the prostitute

Whatever your actual views on men paying for sex, playing the role of a prostitute is another common female fantasy. The very act of being paid for sex means that you are being rewarded for looking gorgeous and someone finding you sexy and desirable. Very often this fantasy takes place in a street or a private club where men have the choice of the women that they want to pay for – and you are the chosen one, deemed sexier than all the others. It's also a chance to fantasise about wearing revealing, tight and seriously suggestive clothes and make-up.

Threesomes and group sex

Now we're definitely entering better-kept-to-a-dream territory. Most men and many women have a threesome fantasy – if you enjoy sex, why wouldn't you want two people pleasuring you simultaneously? And what guy doesn't want to watch two women pleasuring each other? It's hot, exciting and very risqué. But it's also very risky to a relationship. Truth is, as much as a man might fantasise about or even suggest a threesome, he would probably prefer a threesome where neither of the two women (and it's nearly always two women!) are his partner. It's a whole lot less complicated that way.

Having a threesome, or a *ménage à trois*, can open up a Pandora's box of emotions that can be very hard to deal with after the fun is over. There's jealousy, a lack of trust, resentment as well as inadequacy – why weren't you 'good' enough on your own in the first place?

When we're young and at college, after a few too many drinks or a bit stoned, a threesome can seem like an uncomplicated laugh – the sort of sexual experimentation that seems like harmless fun and part of growing up.

But when we're in any kind of a settled relationship, however wild our sex lives might be, a threesome can really threaten the stability of that relationship. This is when the fantasy is generally much better than the reality. It can make you feel self-conscious and under pressure to perform but most importantly it leaves a bitter taste in the mouth, unless – which in itself is rare – you're both absolutely up for it, happy with emotionless sex and strong enough to deal with the guilt, jealousy and blame that so often follows on.

But although I really think (hey, it's just an opinion – albeit one shared by most sexperts) that it's not a great idea to go through with a threesome in real life, there will be those of you out there determined to have a go, so if you must, these are my five basic rules you should be following:

- Agree on the male-to-female combo and who should be involved. This is one instance where strangers are a much better option than friends. There are plenty of swinging options on internet sites where you can keep it relatively anonymous and use a hotel room or an organised club, rather than take it into your own bedroom. And if you're finding your third person online, meet first to discuss what you want out of the situation. And use your instincts to walk away if there's anything remotely dodgy about it or if you just don't see the sexual chemistry working.

- Agree on what's allowed and what isn't. Don't feel that discussing it first somehow diminishes any of the excitement you're going to enjoy. It's absolutely imperative that you discuss what and what isn't allowed, who is allowed to do what to whom and if one of you wants to stop at any point, you all agree to stop. You have to be comfortable with each other's needs and respect each other's limits. Threesomes don't have to involve penetrative sex, for example – the limits just need to be agreed by all parties beforehand.

- Always use a condom. Or a number of condoms, making sure that you change them between partners.

- Make sure your partner is key to the threesome and this is a joint activity with your partner being the focus of attention, not the third party. However much the other person arouses you, you're going home as a couple.

- Don't be too greedy (given that threesomes are pretty much all about greed). When you're not all flailing about doing things to each other, be patient and take it in turns to watch while the other 'couple' get it on.

Animal fantasies

Our wild erotic nature may emerge in animal fantasies. Don't worry, having animal sex fantasies doesn't (usually) mean you want to have sex with animals in real life. You may just revel in the ultra-taboo, bestial wildness. Horses and dogs figure commonly in men's bestiality fantasies, which usually involve them submissively receiving sex from the animal or voyeuristically watching a woman engaged in sex with the animal. Female fantasies tend to involve the woman being the animal, often something in the wildcat family such as a lioness, tiger or cheetah.

Of course, real-life bestiality is appalling to most people. But animal sex fantasies connect you to your primeval nature, offering liberation and freedom from your day-to-day world and your conscious anxieties and burdens as well as releasing any sexual repression that might lie in your subconscious.

Spanking and whipping

Spanking is the kind of fantasy that involves domination (as the spanker) or submission (as the one being spanked). And it's a contentious fantasy because it implies either wanting to be hurt or wanting to hurt someone you care for. And why would you want to do that to your lover? Men especially find the whole spanking issue a bit of a conundrum as it can seem degrading to their partner even if they tell them they like it or want them to do it! So mix the pain–pleasure principle up with some guilt about the role men and women adopt in 'civilised' society and you've got a great recipe for the forbidden pleasure that is the spanking fantasy . . .

A word of warning about spanking. While you might want to turn your fantasy into a reality by giving your partner a swift smack on their bottom – or receiving one yourself – as regularly as you like, using paddles, whips and other paraphernalia (see p. 170) is something else altogether and these props are designed to inflict stinging pain – it's the point of them really – so tread warily until you find your own and your partner's pain threshold.

Sadism and masochism

Sadism and masochism – or just sadomasochism – is commonly known as S & M and is a grittier, more painful and more full-on activity than bondage and domination. It's like advanced bondage and often involves seriously strange and scary paraphernalia like gimp masks and vicious-looking nipple clamps. If bondage and spanking games are soft porn, then S & M 'proper' is like hardcore porn and less than 10% of couples who enjoy bondage games go onto the more serious side of sadomasochism.

Basically, sadism involves inflicting pain on others to feel aroused while masochism is the pleasure you get from pain being inflicted on you by your partner. But there's also a darker side of S & M involving extreme power and domination – which it has in common with bondage games but it tends to be more intense in equipment, practice and fervour. It can also be quite toxic and addictive, so if you find your sex life veering further into using pain for pleasure and you don't feel comfortable about it, it's time to communicate your feelings with your partner. Like any other form of 'kinky' sex practice, its pleasure is almost entirely dictated by trust, communication and honesty.

At its best, S & M can be quite glamorous and panto-mime-like, and if you fancy a journey into its possibilities then either invest in a few of the more bizarre-looking bits of kit offered on many websites or go along to an established and reputable fetish club, like The Torture Garden (details of events can be found at www.torturegarden.com). Everyone dresses up and it can be a fabulous visual feast if nothing else.

Watersports

Watersports, also known as golden showers, is the act of peeing on your partner, or having them pee on you. Its correct term is *urolagnia,* from the Greek combining urine and *lagneia,* meaning lust. The most common form such play takes is for one partner to pee in such a way that the other partner can see and/or feel the golden shower of urine.

Curiously many people find watersports to be one of the most taboo areas of sex play. Given that peeing is a wholly natural and necessary act and that urine itself is virtually sterile, it's surprising it's not more common-place in our repertoires.

It's best done when your bladder is full, obviously, and can be done while standing or sitting over the toilet, while your partner sits down with their legs open, with the aim, literally, of peeing directly on to his penis or her vagina. It can also be done in the bath – or pretty much anywhere where you can clean up easily enough.

It's more common for men to have this fantasy and it is usually the case of being peed on by a woman, rather than the other way around, that dominates this fantasy. Psychoanalytically it may indicate an early contempt or shame about a man's mother, turning the hostility he once felt for one woman into receiving it from another.

Anal sex

I once saw a very funny comedian who was sending up man's desire for anal sex. Why would they want to go to that dry and dirty place when there's a warm, moist, more yielding place just adjacent? It made the women laugh out loud, but most of the men squirmed with uncomfortable acknowledgement. Many men love the anal sex fantasy, because it's such a forbidden area and because it's such a highly erotic zone on their own body, where the prostate gland, or G-spot, is situated. It's also the stuff of a lot of porn films and as such often depicts the powerful man, fully in control, dominating his lover on the pain–pleasure axis of taboo that can be so pleasurable.

Research has shown that around 35% of heterosexual couples have tried anal sex and around half of them continue to do it pretty regularly. But it's still something that many women don't want to try for the obvious reasons – your anus is smaller, tighter and drier than your vagina and you're meant to poo out of it, not have sex with it. And yet most women have met a guy who really wants to try anal sex and has pestered her to do it. And there are men out there who are not beyond trying the 'whoops, wrong hole' trick during sex. If this has happened to you, you'll know that a sharp, penetrative and clumsy thrust into your unlubricated bottom is way more pain than pleasure!

But men – and, to a degree, women – continue to fantasise about anal sex and the truth is that if done properly many women enjoy anal sex. Your rectum being penetrated can be a really pleasurable 'full' feeling, especially if your man can use his finger inside your vagina and/or on your clitoris too. The secret to enjoyable anal sex lies in patience and preparation. You need to use a silicone-based lube – and plenty of it. The sphincter muscles in the anus are like one of the old-fashioned tea-towel holders in reverse and are meant for pushing things *out*, not pushing them in, so it's essential to feel as relaxed as possible and the woman should get her partner to use his fingers to gently soften the muscles first. It often feels uncomfortable at first – whether it's his fingers or his penis – as it feels as if there is an obstructive ridge to pass through before it becomes more comfortable. That's why relaxing – both emotionally and physically – is so important and helps this process along. And whether you're squeamish or not, anal sex is always more pleasant if you have a freshly showered bottom. Even so, anal sex is a breeding ground for sexually transmitted infections, so using a condom is always a good idea.

The most comfortable positions for anal sex are doggy style or missionary – with the woman's knees pulled back and her feet on her lover's shoulders. He should put lubrication on his penis and the woman's anus and proceed with short, slow and gentle thrusts. It's really important that the sphincter muscles are relaxed as if they seize up it can become painful again. Communicate with your partner at all times and don't have high expectations, especially if this is your first time, as it can often take a few attempts to allow your partner to fully penetrate.

Some women find that having an orgasm before anal sex helps relax their sphincter muscles, while others use desensitising anal cream. Frankly, although this numbs the pain it also numbs the pleasure and if it's really hurting too much, it's a sign to stop before you do any internal damage – and disguising that with a desensitising cream is not a good idea.

An alternative to anal sex is to use a butt plug (see page 139). These have flared ends (so they can't disappear inside you) and leave your lover's hands to get on with other stuff. Get your lover to apply some silicone-based lubrication to both the plug and the rim of your anus. If he or she gently pushes the plug, your bottom should suck in the plug a little – they don't go too far in. You simply leave it there and enjoy having sex any other which way. If it isn't inserted at just the right depth, it can feel uncomfortable, so it might not be for you.

Another newer alternative is to use anal beads (see page 140). These special beads are designed to take advantage of the pleasant sensations that can occur as your sphincter muscles open and close around a series of small round objects. These beads, which might be even sized, or graduated in size, are spaced along a stalk or a cord. They are gentler than a butt plug and create a different kind of sensation because when the beads are inserted the sphincter muscles contract and then relax around each individual bead. Pulling them out during an orgasm can really heighten the sensation too.

If anal sex isn't for you – or even if it is – you might enjoy rimming. Rimming is oral anal stimulation and involves thrusting your stiff tongue into the anal passage, as if it were a penis. Or you could just try licking around the area with your tongue and flicking it in and out of the opening. The anus is rich with nerve endings and this in itself can bring a lot of unexpected pleasure for both partners.

Rape fantasies

Forced sex is a very common female fantasy. While it is absolutely nothing to worry about, it is obviously one of the main fantasies that we would *not* want turning into a reality. What it does allow is free range to our imagination to enjoy wild, uninhibited sex without any shred of guilt. While women's fantasies about having sex against their will are usually passionate and dramatic, they are rarely disgusting or unpleasant. It's usually the big burly man taking us on command and is often a way of relinquishing the control that we choose to have – or are obliged to adopt – in our real lives. Alternatively, if we don't have controlling positions in our real lives or feel that we would like to assume more, professionally or personally, fantasising about being the dominant partner and forcing a man to have sex with us is a way of releasing those feelings in a safe and managed way.

Of course, being raped is in actuality one of women's worst fears. And it's why the word rape, with all its dreadful connotations, is not a good word to use for fantasies about having sex against our will. 'Safe rape' or the lovely word 'ravishment' used in the BDSM world might make it a more acceptable fantasy. In a safe rape fantasy, women are given the additional pleasure of resistance and the absolution of guilt, as she didn't ask for this to happen. It's a common fantasy among sexually repressed women (and it's indeed just this type of innocent, inexperienced woman that a man traditionally has fantasies about ravaging) and those women that lack sexual self-confidence. It offers up a higher level of sexual self-confidence because your rapist has clearly found you too desirable to resist.

Rape fantasies often involve women having the most amazing orgasm after being whisked off to some four-poster bed by a tall, dark and dominant stranger, powerless to protest. However, women also fantasise about being raped by an unappealing-looking bloke in the back of a van on a dirty blanket. Whatever the detailed scenario of the fantasy, it allows women to be wild, uninhibited and explore the deepest recesses of their sexual imagination.

So, let's be clear here – fantasising about rape doesn't mean that you want to be raped at all. It's likely that you may have felt very passive in childhood, and the experience of someone dominating you, or sorting out your life for you, is pleasurable. Or you may feel a certain degree of guilt about your sexual desire, whether you're consciously aware of this or not, and in the rape fantasy you are able to abandon yourself to another's needs, appetites and desires – essentially absolving yourself of any responsibility.

Top 10 Female Fantasies

Generally speaking, women's fantasies tend to have a story behind them, rather than getting straight to the sex. Here are the most common ones:

• Sex with another man other than your partner
• Something 'naughty' and new
• Sex with another woman
• 'Rape' – having sex against your will
• Sex with a stranger
• Playing the prostitute
• Being tied up and out of control
• Mills & Boon world
• Sex with a work colleague
• Sex with your current partner

Top 10 Male Fantasies

Men's sex fantasies tend not to be that different from those of women, although they tend to be more carnal than romantic. They often involve quite specific 'naughty' things like anal or oral sex, rather than just something that they might not feel ready to indulge in in real life.

- Sex with another woman other than your partner
- Sex with your current partner
- Sex with a work colleague
- Sex with a stranger
- Watching and being watched during sex
- Anal sex
- Bondage
- Oral sex
- Threesomes
- Being seduced by an older woman

FANTASY SEX AND YOUR STAR SIGN

Given that the conscious or semi-conscious world of fantasies and the subconscious realms of dreams are so closely related, the nature and direction of our fantasies is often in part dictated by our birth sign and the characteristics associated with our astrological chart. So, for some fun – and because I have dealt in some depth with the psychological, deeper meaning of a number of fantasies – see if you recognise your own, or your partner's, fantasies in these signs of the Zodiac.

Aquarius: 21 January–18 February
As an air sign, Aquarians tend to be highly creative and experimental in their sexual fantasies. Being natural communicators, they are often uninhibited

about sharing their fantasies with their partner, encouraging role play where appropriate. Aquarians are built for the pleasure principle, so if something is likely to please them, their imaginations know no bounds. However, they are highly loyal and caring, so fantasies that involve other people, rather than just their partners, are not somewhere that an Aquarian's mind tends to go.

Pisces: 19 February–20 March
As a highly emotional water sign, Pisceans also tend to be playful, creative and often unrealistic about life. They, of all the signs, indulge themselves in all sorts of fantasies from the naughty to the sensual. While they may be very private, even shy, in their day-to-day lives, they come to life during their sexual fantasies, which can be bold and challenging. Pisceans have a huge appetite for sex and due to their high levels of creativity can get bored with repetitive sexual activities, so fantasies are a great way for them to let off some steam. They are also great pleasers – and are happy to go along with dominant or submissive fantasies equally, depending on what their partner prefers.

Aries: 21 March–20 April
As a fire sign, Arians love fantasies about chasing and hunting. They like to capture their partner and often

have fantasies about showing their partner just how great they are in the bedroom – they are keen to prove their sexual prowess and often have the stamina that goes with that. They are open-minded and enjoy experimentation and eroticism. Their fantasies are usually grounded rather than ethereal and they tend to prefer to be the dominant, rather than the submissive, partner.

Taurus: 21 April–21 May
The earthy Taurean can be an exciting and playful lover. Their fantasies tend to be seductive, intense and deliciously slow. They see sex as a physiological as well as a psychological release and want to savour every moment, so their fantasies can be higher on build-up than on action. But as a lover, what they might lack in adventure they more than make up for during foreplay. Ambience is important to them and even male Taureans will make sure that both their fantasies and role play are well prepared for with scented candles, mood music and other props and accessories. Taurus is one appealing package, full of surprises and fun.

Gemini: 22 May–21 June
Geminis love variety and experimentation. A sign that can get bored with routine sex, they fantasise more than most other signs of the Zodiac. But these

fantasies can be quite graphic and the more dominant or urgent fantasies appeal to them most. They are thrill seekers and need to use their imaginations, often wanting to turn them into a reality too. They may seem to lack tolerance and are always in search of the perfect partner to share the perfect fantasy.

Cancer: 22 June–22 July

Another highly emotional water sign, Cancerians like nothing more than to please their lover. Highly emotional, their fantasies tend to be intuitive and nurturing – they are more often the giver in their imaginations, yet tend to prefer more gentle sexual fantasies than other signs. They are romantic, often dismissing fantasies that simply involve sex for emotionally driven scenarios based on love and spirituality as much as the physical acts themselves.

Leo: 23 July–23 August

Leo is one of the feistiest of the fire signs. They like nothing more than completely letting go and savouring every moment of wildness and excitement. They love fast-moving, adventurous fantasies full of action and arousal. They can be vain, often fantasising about how their sexual prowess impresses their partner. They prefer to dominate, rather than be submissive, but providing they can take it to extremes they are also happy to be your slave. They like to cut to the chase, and often are not so keen on the costumes and planning that role play involves, preferring to go straight to the action!

Virgo: 24 August–22 September
Tender and sensitive, Virgoans are perfectionists. They like complete fantasies – imaginary stories that have a beginning, middle and an end. Dreamy and sensual, they can be liberal lovers – but their fantasies tend to be on the safer side of the spectrum. Of all the star signs, Virgo is most likely to repress or even feel guilt about their sexual fantasies, but with a little encouragement and seduction, this rather private sign can fantasise along with the best of them.

Libra: 22 September–23 October
Librans can be passionate and wild lovers – and the breadth of their sexual fantasies is no exception. Like Leos they tend to be almost aggressive in their sexual fantasising and definitely imagine themselves in the more dominant roles, with their partner worshipping them for their sexual expertise. They can be quite materialistic and ambitious too – so often fantasise about scenarios in which they are rich, glamorous and beautiful, or their partners are.

Scorpio: 24 October–22 November
Scorpios are generally considered to be one of the sexiest signs and are powerful and hungry in their sexual appetites. Unsurprisingly, their fantasies are often wild, even extreme. They tend to have the most consistently high libido of any star sign and are probably the most uninhibited. They may see no reason as to why any fantasy that they have could not be fulfilled, so being with a Scorpio lover is not for the faint-hearted! Sensual, passionate and erotic, they fantasise regularly and tirelessly with maximum variation.

Sagittarius: 23 November–21 December
Sagittarians are one of the least emotional signs of the Zodiac, at least where sexual fantasies are concerned. They find it easy to separate love from sex and enjoy fantasies with no emotional ties, such as sex with a stranger. They enjoy eroticism in all its forms and tend to be liberated and adventurous fantasists. They also love to communicate and share knowledge and particularly enjoy spicing up their fantasies – and indeed role play and real-time sex – with some dirty talk.

Capricorn: 22 December–20 January
Capricorns can seem quite straitlaced, but beneath that cool exterior lies a passionate and sexually

adventurous lover. They tend to be more adept lovers when actually in love with their partners, but their sexual fantasies can be quite the reverse – graphic and erotic. They relish control in their fantasies, but also like to be controlled too. The most important thing is that they are able to switch their fantasy lives on and off – coming most to life and having more lurid fantasies when they are actually in the stability of a loving relationship.

In the next chapter, we'll look at the most healthy fantasies that can be adapted and brought to life by role play.

2 Role Play

This is where fantasies become reality. It's the next step up from just imagining what it would be like to actually playing out your fantasies with costumes, props and lots of acting. It's the part where you get the opportunity to let your partner share playing doctors and nurses, rather than just imagining what your cute GP would really be like if he asked you to slip your clothes off and lie down. All you need is your imagination, a sense of humour and a naughty streak. This is very sexy, very private Am Dram. Lots of role play involves very traditional, slightly dated gender roles – doctors and nurses, for example – or involves one partner being dominant or submissive in a way that wouldn't be acceptable or desirable in everyday life. But then that's the point really . . .

Role play is most suitable when you're ready to take

your sexual relationship into new avenues for exploration. There's something about the guise of being in character that allows couples to open their mind to things they might not have considered before. Role playing also makes it easier to reveal some of your hidden desires. It can alleviate some of the boredom and pressure to be creative or try every position under the sun. If this is something you'd like to try, or you'd just like to get new ideas for acting out role-play scenarios, it's always good to prepare a little first – both in terms of your relationship readiness and your props and accessories cupboard.

And just like any other theatrical production, a little planning helps things move along more smoothly and enjoyably.

Set Your Scene

Think about what you want to do and where best to do it. Want to play French maid? Set the scene in the dining room. Fancy your man as a really handy handyman? Have him go outside and knock on the door for his appointment, before you start the action. Whatever you choose it's always better to start the role play when you enter a room or sit down, rather than just try to suddenly begin – which will probably have you both in fits of giggles at how unnatural it feels! Or take your role play away from home – in the garden, on the beach or in a hotel room.

Props

It's much more fun and easier to get into the role if you equip yourselves with some props and costumes. It also gives your partner a visual feast and allows them to actually believe that you are someone else during your role play. Buy, hire or put together an appropriate outfit. Wigs are also great, especially if you're role playing a schoolgirl, judge or similar. And props – whether it's a toy stethoscope, a cat-o'-nine-tails whip or a handyman's toolbox – all add to the atmosphere and 'reality'.

Whatever specific dressing-up props you choose, this is a list of the ten essential props that you should have in your role-play toy box at all times:

- **Lubricant:** whether you feel that you are naturally 'wet' or not – and this can vary due to your age, hormones and libido – there is no doubt that a good water-based lube can make everything more delicious, silky and slippery.

- **Pillows/cushions:** these are a quick and easy addition to role play. If you're planning on getting into some steamy positions, then a good pillow or two can make it a whole lot more comfortable. You can also buy special sex pillows – these are extra firm, offering support in a variety of sexual positions, and are especially good on a wooden floor.
- **Blindfolds:** you can use anything to hand like a scarf, a stocking, a tie or an airline eye mask. Or treat yourself to one of the lovely blindfolds available on the market. By depriving yourself – or your partner – of the power of sight, the sensations of touch, taste, hearing and smell become all the more acute.
- **Handcuffs:** whether you choose some gentle furry or velvety handcuffs or a pair of more heavy-duty steel handcuffs – or perhaps a combination of both depending on the kind of games that you want to play – these restraints are a great way to enhance simple domination and submission games.
- **Paddle:** depending on how into your BDSM games you are (see p. 97), you might want to have a selection of spanking toys – a whip, a paddle, a cat-o'-nine-tails or a riding crop. Because of its wide, flat 'spanking surface', a paddle is one of the most predictable and least scary of the products out there.

- **Stockings and suspenders:** is there a man out there who isn't turned on by a woman in sheer black stockings? A sexy corset or suspender belt and sheer or fishnet – not opaque or hold up – black stockings are very suggestive and an integral part of many of the costumes that women will want to wear during role play.

- **High heels:** there's no point in investing in some silky stockings if you're going to wear a pair of flats with them! A pair of black skyscraper heels is an absolute essential for that leg-lengthening turn-on. High heels are so frequently eroticised in society that not only do they arouse a man, but many women feel sexier, more confident and more empowered when they wear them.

- **Bondage tape:** for when you don't want to use handcuffs, self-sticking bondage tape, which comes in a variety of colours, can be used to wrap ankles, wrists and even bodies!

- **Ostrich feathers:** whether you choose to have a full-on ostrich feather boa or just a few individual feathers, these are one of the softest, most sensuous props to use when role playing.

- **Candles:** have to be one of the easiest ways of casting a flattering and sexy light on just about any role-play game, except perhaps some of the steamier, rough-and-tumble scenarios. A few strategically placed tealights will do or a scented votive or candle in a glass. You can also buy the loveliest natural soft massage candles, where you can combine the light, scent and a tactile thrill! Jimmyjane do some gorgeous massage candles in atmospheric and romantic fragrances like ginger and date, honeysuckle and clover and truffle and gardenia.

Attitude

Whatever characters you choose to adopt in your role play, you will need to think through the role and get yourself in the mood. Is your character innocent and sweet, dominating and stern or prim and posh? Try talking in the kind of voice that suits your character and use your body language to really feel the part. Give your character an appropriate name so that you can use it in your acting. One important thing to remember: role play, especially when one or the other of you is fully in the zone, can get a little steamy and during certain scenarios become more painful than you'd like or cause you distress. You must agree a 'stop' word between you. A word that can't get confused with anything you're doing like 'yes', 'more' or 'harder'. These words are just the kind of expressions that you might find yourself using when involved in a steamy role-play session. Agree a word like 'marmite' or 'radio' – anything that can be heard loud and clear if it all gets a bit too much for you. And don't be afraid to use it. Role play can, and hopefully will, transport you into another world – but it needs to be one of pleasure not distress. Also ask yourself whether you want to be the one in charge of the action or the one dressing up. The majority of role-play scenarios (see dressing up, pp. 94–97) tend to involve the woman getting her kit on, but I've also added a few suggestions for when you want to see your man get into costume, as this can be even more fun!

Role-play Tricks of the Trade

And just like setting the scene, props and the right attitude are essential to the best role-play sessions, there are various little tricks and devices that can be used, as you please, to spice up a variety of scenarios:

- **Talking dirty**
  Hopefully you're already communicating about sex, telling each other what you like – and don't like – and how and what you could do to make it feel even better. Learn to up the stakes during role play, but go gently

at first. Ask him to put his finger inside you or to spank your bottom. And then introduce a few naughty words and phrases of your choice to notch things up a bit. Become a slut, a whore or a virgin. Think porn movie and tell him what a huge, hard, juicy cock he has and what you want to do with it. Keep your voice sexy and low and encourage more dirty talk by asking your partner how it feels, how wet or horny they're feeling and if they want more or want it harder or faster.

- **Sensory deprivation**
Sensory deprivation is where you limit or impair one or more of your five senses – touch, hearing, smell, taste or vision – in order to enhance one or more of the other senses as a result. Sensory deprivation is incredibly arousing to some people, so bondage gear such as blindfolds and masks that cover the eyes and mouth work really well during role play.

- **Leather and PVC**
What is it about leather and PVC that makes us think of sex? Almost all fetish and bondage clothes are made of leather, rubber or PVC and even those who forego BDSM find wearing something tight, sculpted and black makes them feel sexier. Much of it has to do with base animal instincts – the sense of wild, unabated sexiness by wearing or seeing someone wearing such a tight, soft and flexible material that belongs in a non-

human world where sexual mores and niceties don't really exist. It's also plump with promise – the body is usually contained by zips or lacing that beg to be undone and it clings like a second skin leaving nothing to the imagination. Whether your role play includes full fetish gear or just an occasional leather or faux leather prop, it definitely adds more than a spark of wickedness to the proceedings.

FOOD IN ROLE PLAY

Food and sex have always been inextricably linked. Both arouse all our five senses of sight, touch, taste, smell and hearing, and all are physically linked in the limbic system of the brain, which controls our emotional attitude and activity. Adventurous eaters and those who savour flavour often make exciting, sensual lovers, while fussy, fast eaters on a limited diet tend to be less hungry in the bedroom too . . .

Eating and making love both involve anticipation, expectation and fulfilment. Good food is often a prelude to good sex. And both food and sex touch us in a deep and emotional way.

Research has clearly shown people who enjoy their food and are willing to experiment are much more likely to savour a good lovemaking or role-play session, whereas those who are parsimonious about food or unwilling to try anything new will tend to follow suit sexually. And then there is the terminology of eating and food that is heavily linked with sex. Nibbling, biting, sucking, swallowing, licking and tasting are all words that lend themselves easily to both pleasures.

Good lovers prepare good food for their partners. They pay attention to colour, visual appearance and presentation and seductive aromas. In role-play terms, food lends itself to all sorts of scenarios that involve feeding frenzy orgies or simple sensuous foods – like strawberries dipped in chocolate – that are ripe, delicious and oozing sex appeal.

In Greek mythology certain fruits, such as **figs**, **grapes** and **pomegranates** were used to represent sexual union, virility and fertility. Red and pink foods are often used in a sexual sense as they remind us of both the mouth and the lips of the vagina. Wearing red lipstick or lipgloss to look sexy has the same roots.

Oysters are the classic aphrodisiac food, of course. They happen to contain more zinc than any other foodstuff, which a man needs to increase his testosterone level and sperm production. But it's also curiously primeval and stimulating to eat a live food, still in its own juices. As Hugh Fearnley-Whittingstall put it so brilliantly: 'A slippery, salty oyster, recumbent and ready inside its glistening, pearl-lined cavity, is undeniably arousing.'

Truffles are another luxury food that are said to have aphrodisiac qualities. This time it's the aroma that is sexy, rather than the texture or the taste. They are heavy and musky and replicate the pheromones that make us sexually aroused. **Chocolate** is another favourite. Apart from the fact that it releases the feel-good chemicals, endorphins, into our body, it is also one of the few foodstuffs that melts at body temperature.

Then there are some odd ones, of course. The **durian** fruit from East Asia – highly pungent and foul-smelling – is also said to be an aphrodisiac. There is a saying in Asia that 'When the durian comes in, the sari goes up'!

One of the reasons that the pleasures of food and sex are so deeply linked is the make-up of our mouth and tongue. The lips and tongue are packed with ultra-sensitive nerve endings, and kissing – just like good food, well cooked and delicious to taste – makes our blood pressure and our pulse rate increase, as well as our pupils dilate. Just like sex . . . So choosing to include finger foods and aphrodisiacs into your own role play can be both seductive and exciting and one of the most truly sensuous 'props' that you can use.

Dressing Up

Role play simply wouldn't be the same without accessorising with appropriate outfits and props. You can choose to spend anything from a few quid on a basic role-play costume from a fancy dress shop or mail order company to several hundred pounds on a complete, ready-made – and, at the upper end of the price scale, fully customised – outfit of your choice.

Unless you're seriously into any one form of role play – like dressing up in a velvet-and-lace burlesque costume or a full leather bondage kit or can't imagine wanting to be anything other than a cowgirl or a French maid – there isn't much point in investing a fortune. Use your imagination and you'll find that in a few versatile props – like a feather boa and a blindfold – plus a wig or two are probably all you need. And in fact much of the point of successful and fulfilling role play is not to return to the same roles and scenarios over and over again, but to regularly try something new to maximise your pleasure and keep your sex life vibrant, varied and fresh.

But it's always good to have inspiration and to know what is out there – so that you can buy a complete outfit if you wish or use the descriptions below to help you adapt and collect your own.

I've trawled some of the better websites (so that you don't have to!) and, while this is by no means a definitive list of the dressing-up/full costume end of role play, it gives some variety and food for further thought. As ever, most of the costumes are for women. There are just a few outfits for men out there and most are hugely unsexy and very predictable – so if you want to dress up your partner, or you're a guy who fancies getting into kit, you'll have to use a little more of that essential prop known as your imagination!

Women

Bunnygirl: fluffy ears, tail and wrist cuffs, leotard or corset, black bow tie

Policewoman: black minidress, peaked cap, cop badge, truncheon, handcuffs

Little angel: white satin minidress, fingerless gloves, feathered angel wings, feather halo

Horny little devil: red minidress, matching thong, devil horns and tail

Alice in Wonderland: gingham puffed-sleeved dress, white apron, headband, over-the-knee socks or white stockings

Wicked witch: little black dress, pointy hat, cape

French maid: puffed-sleeved black dress, white apron, lace choker, lace garter, mop cap, feather tickler/duster

Air stewardess: pencil skirt, blouse, air-hostess hat, scarf

Sailor girl: little white button or zip-up dress, navy scarf, sailor hat

Army girl: combat kit – camouflage dress or shorts, army cap, belt holder with bullets, toy gun

Miss Whiplash: one-piece zip-up PVC black catsuit, whip

Sexy secretary: pinstriped minidress, suspenders and stockings, glasses, necktie, thong

Cowgirl: cute minidress, cowgirl hat, checked scarf

Sexy flapper: loose sequinned dress, feather boa, sequinned headband, string of pearls

Naughty nurse: short white button-down or zip dress, nurse's cap, stethoscope

Pirate: minidress, velvet jacket, skull and crossbones hat, belt, eyepatch

Sexy schoolgirl: miniskirt, white blouse, necktie, straw boater, over-the-knee socks or stockings

Men

Sexy stripper: bow tie, cuffs, thong pants

Hot surgeon: shorts, mask, hat, gloves, stethoscope

Horny handyman: mechanic's boiler suit, spanner, drill, screwdriver

Fireman: all-in-one brown and yellow jumpsuit, matching hard hat

Pirate: velvet lace-up shirt, bandanna, boot covers, belt, cuffs, eyepatch

Sexy biker: black waistcoat, matching trousers, hat, choker, boot covers

Bondage Play

I've called this bondage play because most of the stuff that I talk about in this section is pretty much what you'll want to 'play' at home, rather than in an environment, like a dungeon, specifically built for the diehard fans. Many role-play games, like fantasies, are covered by what is commonly known as BDSM (bondage, domination, submission and masochism). It's naughty enough and involves one of you being submissive (a sub) while the other is dominant (a dom). It involves a certain degree of pain and includes whipping, spanking, tying up and scratching. But it can be sexy and fun during role play – owing more to leather, high heels and silk than to the gimp suits, ball gags and chains of more serious BDSM enthusiasts. It's highly arousing because it increases sexual tension in the nicest way – being at the mercy of someone else (or doing the controlling) when they are teasing, licking or penetrating you is exciting, edgy and wholly *not* what we do in everyday life. Causing pain, expecting servitude and physically restraining your partner: these activities do not make up a healthy relationship on a day-to-day basis!

The pain–pleasure threshold, on which all bondage play is based, can be an overwhelming sensation that can boost the intensity of your orgasms to new levels, due to the brain releasing feel-good chemicals called endorphins to help reduce the pain caused by a spank or slap. You may also enjoy seeing a temporary mark left on your lover's bottom or thigh due to the punishment you have meted out. Whipping, slapping or spanking your partner's bottom, thighs or legs will also heighten the nerve endings in the targeted area, making your lover's skin much more responsive to stroking, licking, biting, nibbling and scratching after it has been struck with a whip or paddle.

Bondage itself is the act of tying up your partner (or them tying you up) so that they are helpless, writhing and in your sexual control and command. You have the opportunity to act as the dominant partner – doing the tying – or the submissive partner at your lover's mercy. While the physical act of bondage – tying up your partner with bondage tape, a silk scarf or handcuffs, for example – is a major turn-on, the verbal form of bondage is just as exciting. Commanding your lover, or being told what to do by your lover, is an intensely sexy feeling that will lead you to do and command things you might normally be too embarrassed to mention. You can use bondage to act out role-play scenarios (such as those mentioned on pp. 101–26) or to pull apart or spread open parts of your lover's body. You can tie your partner to a chair, a bed or just use it to restrict normal movement.

- **Being a great dom**
  - Be demanding and commanding – this is not a time to be polite.
  - You must threaten punishment and then carry it out.
  - Tease them to please them – unpredictability makes bondage play even sexier.

- **Being a great sub**
  - You must be subservient and obedient at all times, unless you want to be punished.
  - You must be polite and express gratitude at all times – before, during and after punishment.
  - Make sure your body language reflects your servility – kneel down, look adoringly at your partner or stay on all fours.

BONDAGE ESSENTIALS

Trust is an important tool in bondage play, so make sure that you stick to the following points:

- **always remember your chosen 'stop' word**
- **don't tie someone up for too long**
- **be aware that your partner might get anxious or have a panic attack**
- **if your partner says the 'stop' word do just that, however fantastic you're feeling**

Suggested Scenarios

Here are some popular role-play scenarios and some ones of my own. Think of these as keys to unlocking your sexual imagination – go for the ones that turn you and your partner on and then take it from there. Don't follow these scenarios rigidly – they're not scripts – and nor should you stick to the suggested male or female 'roles' if your predilections lead you elsewhere. You and your partner are the ones in control here, so the roles you take and what you say and do – and how – are entirely up to both of you. The most important rule here is to have fun!

Mistress of discipline
The woman should dress in a leather or PVC outfit. Keep it black and disciplinarian – even a satin pencil or leather skirt and black shirt would be good. Make it tight rather than obviously revealing. Black stockings and knee-high black boots are a must. Other accessories include a 'weapon' or two: paddle, belt, hairbrush, whip and wrist restraints. He should be dressed in a normal, casual way. The mistress asks him to undress. Slowly. If he's not doing it to the mistress's satisfaction, she should insist that he tries again or he'll be punished, and should crack her whip a few times to ensure he knows exactly

who is in control – her voice should be low and firm. The mistress is in charge and she can order him to do whatever she wants.

Once he is naked, the mistress could ask him to watch her undress. Or she could command him to lie face down, while he is blindfolded and his hands bound together behind his back. He is not allowed to squirm, writhe or make any sound. If he should even think about trying to move things along at his own pace, the mistress should ensure that he knows that his subordination will be dealt with in a manner of her choice. This is a good time to crack that whip, riding crop or paddle. This is meant to cause some pain but it isn't meant to create weals on his back or his bottom and it's definitely not the time to let rip on any underlying grudges on him.

He'll beg the mistress to stop, but unless he's actually using the chosen 'stop' word (see pp. 88–89) she must carry on. The mistress of discipline will only show him mercy when *she's* so aroused that he's going to have to be untied in order to have that immediate sex that she needs right now!

Props: black pencil skirt, black tightly fitting top, stockings, high-heeled boots, handcuffs, paddle or riding crop.

Sex slave

This time she is the slave and he is the master. He is going to make sure that his partner has the wildest of times and she has to follow his instructions and commands very carefully. She is completely naked – except perhaps for the odd ankle or wrist restraint or blindfold, as he wishes. He'll ask her to do something simple at first – fetch him a drink or stroke his shoulders. Then he gets bolder with his demands and warns his slave that if she doesn't comply, she'll get punished. A few props, like a hairbrush, should be kept within arm's reach, just in case the slave is really naughty and doesn't do as she was asked. He'll tell her that she has been a very bad girl and just when he thinks she might be enjoying his sex play, he'll stop whatever he's doing and move on to something else. Remember that he is completely in control and it's his call as to whether his slave should be experiencing pleasure or not. Like all role play, this should be simple, not-so-clean fun, but if things are getting out of hand, remember to use the chosen 'stop' word (pp. 88–89) before things get too uncomfortable.

Props: blindfold or scarf, handcuffs or bondage tape, hairbrush or paddle.

Who's been a naughty boy/girl then?

Teacher and pupil role-playing games offer endless scope for sexual fun. Once into your chosen character, you can wave goodbye to your inhibitions and let your imagination take you to a world where almost anything is permissible. So lock the bedroom door and prepare for some thrilling and unusual extra-curricular activities.

For this version, if you're a student, you'll need to get yourself kitted up in a simple white shirt and black or grey trouser combo if you're the boy; for a girl a gymslip or school skirt, white blouse, tie and knee socks completes the look, which is a bit St Trinian's – dishevelled, slutty, with more than a promise of naughtiness.

Dressing up as a male teacher is not too difficult – go for a tweedy, academic look, whereas the female teacher can look as saucy as she pleases – tight shirt, blouse unbuttoned just a little too low flashing sexy underwear, high heels and suspenders.

The student is, of course, in some trouble at school and must be appropriately punished by the teacher. Or perhaps the pupil has done especially well at a subject and the teacher wants to show you just how much he appreciates your efforts. Or perhaps the schoolboy or girl has been having trouble with biology, and the teacher can share the benefit of his or her experience with that too.

Here's a more detailed scenario appropriate for a female teacher/male student combination. Of course, reverse and change the roles to suit you. This should be seen as a jumping-off point.

It's a baking hot afternoon and all the other students have gone home. The naughty schoolboy is writing an essay entitled 'Why I must not talk in class', but he would rather be out playing footie with his mates. His rather cute teacher is busy preparing for tomorrow's lessons on the blackboard, when suddenly she drops her chalk. The schoolboy glances up as she bends down to pick it up and catches an inviting glimpse of a smoothly stockinged thigh under her straitlaced clothing.

The schoolboy is quite excited – it's almost worth the detention to have seen such a sight. Lucky for him that she didn't see him looking. She busies herself at the blackboard again and the pupil tries to concentrate on his essay, but it's no longer the thought of his mates playing soccer that's putting him off his stride.

Glancing up again, the student sees that his teacher is writing something at the very top of the blackboard – and her skirt has ridden right up the back of her legs. She's wearing stockings! They're held up by a lacy little suspender belt that she is wearing on top of very brief panties – which leaves little to the imagination.

Suddenly, she turns around and notices that the

schoolboy has been looking at her and she's angry. Simple detention and essay writing will no longer do. The student must be punished more appropriately and given a lesson that he won't forget in a long time . . .

Props: male student – white shirt, black/grey trousers and school tie; female student – grey or navy pleated skirt or gymslip, white school shirt or blouse, tie, white knee socks, big pants – Bridget Jones style! Male teacher: jeans, shirt and tie, tweedy jacket (with leather patches on the elbows, if you can manage it!); female teacher: tight pencil skirt, prim blouse, glasses, stockings, suspenders and lacy panties.

Disco delight

Set up your living room so it resembles a bar or a club – turn down the lights and turn on loud rock music. Get a bottle of wine or champagne with glasses and pour a drink for yourself and your lover. The man can be the one who is just in the club or bar chilling with some friends, or even by himself. In fact, you could even take this out of the house. Arrange to meet in a bar not so far from where you live, and one of you should arrive a few minutes before the other.

The woman plays the role of the very sexy and needy girl looking for a man to tease and fulfil her hot sexual appetite. She sits on a barstool or chair flirting with the man she's noticed – but not being too obvious. She should make good use of her legs, body language and eyes. Of course, it's easy for the roles to be reversed here too – the man could come on to his partner, telling her just what he'd like to do to her.

Let things develop from there. Pretend you don't know each other and you have a choice of not talking and letting two strangers have a night of passion, or let your role play turn into a sexy discussion between two complete strangers. Remember – if you're doing this outside your house, make sure you get home, before things become too heated!

Props: chair or bar stool, wine or champagne, sexy, revealing clothing.

Lady of the manor

This is another opportunity for both partners to get into costume as well as into character. The woman plays a very rich, very posh older woman living in a fabulous country pile – alone, of course, apart from the occasional maid or butler. She dresses accordingly – with her hair piled up into a bun and a smart suit accessorised with a few brooches and a silk scarf (it can be used later as a blindfold!). The male could be the gardener – younger and a bit rough around the edges but always pleased to help out for little money and the privilege of serving the lady of the house.

The woman's lonely, and her very sexy young gardener is working outside, tending her shrubbery in nothing more than a vest and a pair of jeans. She watches as his strong hands tenderly prune her bush and his upper arm muscles ripple and glisten with sweat. Perhaps she wonders what those hands would feel like running over her breasts, so she opens the back door, calls to him and invites him in for a refreshing cup of tea . . .

Props: male – jeans, singlet vest top. Female – smart suit, string of pearls or other formal jewellery, silk scarf.

Sex worker

The woman should arrange to meet her partner on a dark, secluded street corner not too far from her home (in a safe place, for obvious reasons). She's kitted out in some tight, revealing and slutty clothes, stockings and suspenders, perhaps a too-short tight mini and a clashing silky top. She should then put on a big coat and stand around on the corner for a minute or two to get into the feel of the role.

The man should arrive in his car, park a few feet away and watch his partner for a few minutes. Then he should pull up slowly in front of her, lower his car window and ask whether she's available for business and how much she costs. She should then quote him a price. He wants to know what he gets for his money. She opens her coat and shows him exactly what he's going to get for the 'hire fee'. He might accept or they might negotiate for a moment or two, perhaps suggesting a few extras for his trouble. While he drives home, she should keep in businesslike, impersonal character while he tells her what he'd like her to do to him. She then assures him of ultimate customer satisfaction.

Props: cheap, tarty clothes, preferably a size too small, stockings and suspenders, big wrap coat.

Stripper and client

A woman stripping for her man is quite a turn-on for both partners, particularly if she has an exhibitionist streak! But for a shyer woman striptease or lap dancing can be quite a challenge, especially if she is very conscious of her body. Lighting a few candles is a way of enhancing the ambience and softening any harsh light. Or use a red light bulb or cover a lamp in some red, silky material. There is no need to strip completely naked either. She can keep her bra, pants or a corset on or use a sarong or two to cover up, just teasingly showing glimpses of her flesh.

The idea is to tease and tempt. She could use a strategically placed feather boa to tickle her man and gently gyrate using some sexy background music. She should wear a garter so that he can pop a note or two inside it, when he's pleased with what she is doing. Or he could pop a tenner into her bra, belly-dancer style.

A sexy twist on the paid strip scenario is for it to be impromptu and free. For example, the woman sends her man out into the garden to offer him a highly suggestive striptease through the window: he can see her, but can't touch her or get back into the house without her say-so. Make sure your neighbours don't get a free peepshow as well – unless that adds to the frisson of your role play, of course!

Props: sexy, easy-to-remove clothing, feather boa, stockings and suspenders, a garter, candles or red light, skyscraper heels.

Celebrity and fan
This is a scenario where the male/female roles could easily be reversed.

She's worshipped this movie/rock star for years. He's hot, sexy and always in the news. Girls flock around him and he's always seen at the best parties. She's managed to get a backstage pass to see him and has half an hour alone with him in his dressing room. She's looking fabulous – hair and make-up freshly done – and she's not going to let this opportunity pass without ensuring that she takes away some unforgettable memories. As he looks at her and smiles, taking in this gorgeous and sexy woman, their eyes lock and she knows what she has to do. She's going to give him half an hour of the wildest time he's ever had. This is her dream come true and she's not going to waste a moment . . .

Props: sexy clothing, full eye make-up. Maybe a few toys secreted in your handbag to liven things up.

Damsel in distress

This can be anything you and your partner likes – so long as the woman's playing the helpless female. Maybe she's been locked out of her bedroom, wearing nothing but a slinky robe. Maybe her shower needs mending and she's just emerged wearing only a soft towel wrapped round her. Whatever scenario you and your partner choose, keep in character as a woman who simply can't manage without the help of this strong, burly and rather sexy knight in shining armour who has stepped in to help. What would she have done without him? She must express her gratitude in a way that she knows he'll accept as payment for his sterling work.

Props: basic stuff depending on the role. A large bath towel, a silky robe or perhaps nothing but a knowing smile . . .

The librarian

You and your partner can start role playing this in a quiet corner of a bookshop or library, or if you have bookshelves at home use these as props, especially as she reaches up high to get a book from the top shelf, revealing black lacy stocking tops under a prim skirt. Or maybe she'll be bending over to reach a book right over in the corner of the bookcase.

The librarian is efficient, organised and ever so slightly snobby. Her partner is looking for a book that she rather disapproves of (this one perhaps!) and she looks down at him, over her thick-rimmed glasses, with thinly disguised disdain. She is in the business of organising important reference books, not providing salacious reading material for an impertinent young man. She asks him why he would want such a book. He says that he is happy to tell her exactly why and suggests that she might feel a little more relaxed and comfortable by letting her hair down (literally and figuratively!) and removing her glasses, while she sits down next to him on the big squishy sofa in the corner.

Props: pencil skirt, prim blouse, stockings and suspenders, stern glasses, books.

Doctors and nurses

The stuff of old-fashioned romance novels, there are few of us who haven't fantasised about dishy doctors or cute nurses. They have both power and command as well as caring, nurturing qualities. It's a heady combination. And, for many of us, playing 'Doctors and Nurses' while at primary school was our first taste of what it was like to 'flirt' with the opposite sex.

Both of you should dress up as medical practitioners, he as a doctor, in a white coat and a stethoscope, she in a fancy dress nurse's costume or a simple cotton dress and apron dressed up with a nurse's hat, fob watch, black stockings and flat shoes. Or one partner plays the patient who the doctor/nurse asks to go behind the curtain, lie down and remove his or her top so he/she can check the patient's heartbeat. Or she plays a junior nurse with a major crush on the new, handsome and oh-so-shy doctor that's just started working with her. Perhaps he's cross and stern and never notices her because he's married to his career. Or gentle and caring and gives her the occasional lingering glance that makes her blush. Whatever scenario, find some sort of excuse to ensure that the nurse finds a way to get the doctor alone, so that he is in no doubt as to how she feels about him.

Props: male – white lab coat, stethoscope; female – nurse's costume or plain cotton dress and apron, stockings, 'sensible' shoes.

Calling in the expert

She is an experienced woman who has had plenty of lovers and yet none of them has given her the oral sex that she needs and deserves. So she calls in an expert to give her a little more than lip service . . .

There is a knock at the door: it's the silver-tongued gigolo that she ordered earlier. Briefly and formally she beckons him into the living room, hitches up her skirt and spreads her legs widely while sitting astride a comfortable chair or sofa. Of course she has no knickers on – she's paid for a professional service and she doesn't want to waste time removing underwear. She then allows the gigolo to offer her the platinum service – the most delicious and effective mouth and tongue expertise he can imagine.

Props: comfortable chair or sofa.

French maid

One of the most 'traditional' of role plays, there's something quaintly old-fashioned about playing the role of a French maid, so make the most of it – the costume can be easily found at any costume site or shop, or pull something together from your own props cupboard.

He should be dressed beautifully in a dinner jacket and bow tie or in a smoking jacket and cravat. Perhaps his hair is slicked back in the style of the 1920s. She is a sexy little French maid, dressed in a way-too-short black frock, a white lacy apron and a floppy mop cap. Oh and, of course, uber-sexy stockings and suspenders and teeteringly high black shoes. Her aim is to please her master by serving him drinks and food from a silver tray. She is an innocent employee, however naughtily dressed, and she would be shocked to her core if he, her master, were to behave inappropriately with her. Which of course he is just about to do . . .

Food works well in this scenario – the more slippery, juicy and soft the better.

Props: male – dinner jacket, black trousers, dress shirt, bow tie; female – plain little black dress, white apron, mop cap, high heels, serving tray with food and drink.

Roman decadence

Take yourselves on a trip back in time to the most sensual and decadent of all civilisations and partake in the extraordinary physical pleasures of ancient Rome.

The Romans possessed a rich sensuality and an appreciation of physical pleasure that has almost been lost to the modern world. The warm climate, an abundance of fresh and delicate food and plenty of leisure ensured that there was both the time and inclination for love.

Dress flamboyantly in tunics or togas made of gently draped muslin or old sheets. Use coloured scarves and red, gold or purple jewellery to add to the opulence. You can even make a headband of bay leaves!

Make a drama out of the food itself. Romans ate their meals while reclining on couches. This was considered a sign of refinement and social position and is an ideal role-playing scenario to bring in some delicious ripe fruit and other sensuous foods. Go for cheese, cold meats, oysters, savoury biscuits, prawns, smoked salmon – any finger food that will add sensuality and decadence to the occasion. Make sure there is plenty of fresh fruit – peaches, pineapples, pomegranates, passion fruit, figs and, of course, juicy grapes. Serve everything with copious quantities of chilled wine, to drink from goblet-shaped glasses.

Props: togas and tunics made of muslin or sheets. Bright, bold gemstone jewellery to pin and keep the togas in place. Strappy sandals.

Roman baths

You could take the Roman theme one step further by turning your own bathroom into a decadent orgy of Roman pleasure. In the ancient world, the bath was not just a simple means to clean; it was a form of recreation, a way of relaxing and socialising. The humblest citizens could enjoy the pleasures of the huge and cavernous public baths, while the nobility had their very own bathing halls in which to while away the mornings and afternoons.

Your own bathroom is unlikely to be on such a grand scale, but with a few plans and basic preparations you can also indulge yourself and your partner in a languid and sensuous Roman bathing experience. Run a warm bath and sprinkle it liberally with scented oil. Use tea lights around the bathroom to create soft lighting and atmosphere. You could also play some opera music – not exactly Roman, but it will fit the bill musically with its stirring lyrics and opulent extravagance. Take it in turns to soak in the scented, oil-rich water or you can bathe together. Make it a really sensual experience; use large sponges soaked alternately in hot and cold water over each other's skin. Choose natural, traditionally scented soaps and shampoos, with perfume such as aloe vera or sandalwood, and above all take your time, sensuously washing every inch of your partner's body.

Once you're out of the bath, you can lay towels and cushions on the floor and take it in turns to cover each other's body with the scented oil. You can use one of the massage techniques on pp. 176–80. Once your partner's whole body is glistening, take a small, blunt scraper, like an old credit card, and gently scrape all the oil off the body in soft movements in the direction of your heart. This exfoliation should leave the skin tingling and super-smooth.

Props: scented bath oil, massage oil, towels, candles, cushions, blunt scraper, natural shampoos and soap.

Photographer and model

The traditional way of acting out this role play is for the woman to be the model and the man to be the photographer, but as the only rules in role play are the ones you decide for yourselves there is no reason why you shouldn't reverse these roles! The photographer-and-model scenario is perfect for watching each other and acting out fantasies. It can be used to encourage the model to become something he or she may have always wanted to be – a wildcat in front of the camera or a glamour model.

The lighting needs to be right here. While in the real world lighting in a photographic studio tends to be incredibly bright and strong, you don't need to replicate it here. Bright light is a bit intimidating when you want your partner to strip off, so dim the lights or use a few soft lamps instead.

The photographer needs to encourage the model to make love to the camera, so get your partner to be as seductive or as raunchy as he or she feels like. You might want to set the scene right from the start with the photographer offering the model a glass of champagne to get relaxed and in the mood. You might want to incorporate a few props too – a furry blanket or throw and some sexy undies.

The bonus of this role play is that you'll also end up with some photos to remember the scenario by!

Props: camera or mobile phone with flash, champagne, furry throw or blanket, sexy underwear, any other accessories of your choice.

Artist and nude model
Even if neither of you have any artistic inclination at all, you can have a lot of fun with one of you posing as a

nude model while the other sketches what they see. Just make sure you're in a warm room – erect nipples are sexy but shivering while you try to keep still in a cold room isn't! Lie on the sofa, a furry rug or your bed in the most provocative position you can muster and let your partner start to create his or her masterpiece . . .

Painting your naked lover is an interesting experience. Whether you have artistic talent or not, it is an extremely sensual exercise and can be highly erotic and satisfying in itself. It gives the painter a chance to study their lover's form long and hard – and to feast their eyes on every fleshy hollow, mould, angle and crevice that makes up the human body.

The artist can study such things that may have been considered individually but never as a whole – the way the skin tones change, the pattern of hair growth and the way the shadows are cast by the curves or muscles.

Begin with bold, wild strokes to capture the curves and general shape of your partner. Then fill in the detail – by taking in all the details that especially appeal to you. You will be looking at your lover in a new way and may well discover aspects of him or her that seem unfamiliar – a mole here, a patch of darker skin there. It's not that you were inattentive before, simply that now you are paying more attention as you are taking the time to reproduce your lover's body on paper.

Props: the simplest of props is needed here. Blank paper or a sketchbook, pencils or charcoal. Maybe an easel. A rug or blanket. Maybe a boa or a string of pearls draped suggestively to add atmosphere. Artist's beret optional!

Seducing a virgin

The woman should ensure she dresses in prim and proper clothes, a blouse with maybe just a button undone at the neck. Either wear a Doris Day, 1950s-style oh-so-innocent skirt or maybe a pencil skirt. She could wear bare legs, sheer or opaque stockings or even knee socks.

She sits with her partner on the sofa and tells him that she has something to confess. She's reached a certain age and while she's a woman of the world in many ways, there's one thing that hasn't happened to her yet. She's still a virgin and has been searching for the right man to deflower her. This confession works best if it's kept polite and coy, with perhaps a touch of nerves showing. Or, while keeping that sweet and innocent virginal tone, she should tell her lover something really dirty that she'd like him to do to her. He should then explain how gentle – or indeed how rough – he's going to be with her and explain what exactly she's been missing all these years and how he's going to rectify that unfortunate situation. He'll be writhing with desire – but both parties should make sure that the role play is kept going for as long as you both are able to hold all that anticipation in place.

Props: cute and sweet gingham skirt or dress or something vaguely vintage, headband, knee socks and sensible shoes.

Boss and secretary

This scenario revolves around the work situation, and the power exchange that frequently takes place between a woman and her male boss. It is supposed that the boss is in control, but when sex is involved, this is reversed and the woman is actually calling the sexual shots. She loves this because it gives her the power in that particular situation, even if she has very little influence during her working hours.

There are various different mini-scenes that can be created here. She could hide something under the boss's desk – which in reality is your dining table – before he's due to take an important phone call. While he's in the midst of this phone call, she walks slowly, sexily and deliberately up to his desk, kneels down and without saying anything at all, gives him some seriously distracting oral sex. He has to continue with this important phone call without faltering in his speech.

Alternatively, she could play the very sexy secretary

by wearing some daring underwear to 'work' – like stockings and suspenders or crotchless pants. While continuing to undertake her usual duties in the most professional way, and while her boss is engrossed in paperwork or on his computer, she makes sure that he gets a glimpse or two of what she's wearing underneath her rather sober work wear. She might bend over the photocopier or stretch up to reach a file off the shelf, while ensuring that her skirt rides up at the same time.

No touching or talking is allowed until the boss is practically gagging for sex with his naughty secretary.

Props: desk or dining table, chair, office-type clothing, crotchless panties or stockings and suspenders, laptop and phone.

Naughty neighbour

This is a good scenario to play early in the evening just as twilight begins. She'll have come from work and decided to have a long, scented bath to help her unwind. She's just settling down with a good book, a glass of wine and a great CD when there's a knock on the door. Although she's freshly scrubbed and smelling sweet, she's wearing nothing but a silk robe. She decides to see who could be knocking on her door and when she opens it, there is her neighbour wondering if he could borrow a cup of sugar as he seems to have run out. It would be rude to leave him on the doorstep, so she invites him in for a drink. They indulge in a little neighbourly chit chat while she casually lets her robe drop open, so that he can see just what a good (or bad!) neighbour she really could be . . .

Props: wine, music, silky robe and maybe some sexy lingerie.

Horny handyman

Another traditional role-play scenario where the woman can adopt the submissive role of the helpless housewife who, overwhelmed with loneliness, desire and gratitude, can't help but fall into the arms of this man who simply came around to sort out her leaky valve. Or she might want to adopt a dominant stance by taking this young and innocent apprentice plumber and show him a thing or two about how pipe work really functions. Whatever version you choose, he should don a loose boiler suit – great for adding to the atmosphere and dropping in one fell swoop – as well as knocking on her door, toolbox in hand. She should keep her voice low and sexy – even the most simple of tools for the job can sound suggestive and very, very naughty.

Props: boiler suit or casual clothes suitable for manual work, toolbox and tools.

Polo player

On of my personal favourites, this is a very *Officer and a Gentleman* or James Bond scenario and indeed can be played out with your partner as a captain of a cruise liner or an airline pilot. The main thing here is that, unusually for role play, it's the man who really gets to go to town on the dressing up. Suit, epaulettes and cap – whatever it takes to recreate the debonair, powerful and sexy man in charge.

Back to our polo player . . . This role suits a man with rugby player's thighs and a certain presence. She will be dressed in a pretty, floaty dress having decided to go to watch a polo match. She is attracted to one player in particular, with his smart white jodhpurs, bulging biceps and tan, weathered riding boots. How handsome he looks on his horse. But, oh no, he has had a fall and while there is no harm done, he needs to sit down and take a few minutes out. And there he is, sitting on her sofa, sipping a cool, reviving drink, sweat gently glistening on his brow and arms and just a little turf smut on his cheek. His legs are slight open, there's a gentle bulge just to the left of his tight white riding pants and he's thanking her profusely for coming to his rescue . . .

Props: male – tight white trousers or jodhpurs, polo shirt, knee boots; female – summery, floaty dress.

Now that you've seen how games can become fantasy and how fantasy can evolve into role play, let's look in more detail at the huge array of sex toys available that can spice up all aspects of your sex life.

3 Sex Toys

Sex toys come in a bewildering array of shapes and sizes and their uses are not always immediately obvious. Some look like they might cleave you in half or are as small as your lipstick, others look rather beautiful but are hugely expensive while some simply look like you might end up in your local A & E Department! Sex toys of all descriptions are hugely popular: according to a recent sex survey from Durex, more than one in five adults have used a vibrator. And these vibrators don't simply vibrate – they twist and turn, swivel and are designed to be used on your mouth, bottom, breasts, urethra and perineum, and can be used directly on a woman's clitoris and vagina, as well as a man's penis and anus.

The truth is that sex toys (a far better term than the rather unfortunate-sounding 'marital aids' or 'sex aids' as they used to be called!) have been around for centuries. The Ancient Greeks used them and sex toys have been found that are over two thousand years old. And in China, the third-century Han Dynasty created dildos made from ivory and wood, many of which were double ended to accommodate two women at once!

By the mid-nineteenth century dildos were widely used and manufactured. Rather than giving sexual pleasure, they were advertised as medical aids. Medical massage didn't have any stigma and was widely administered as a muscle relaxant and stress reliever.

The first patented steam-powered vibrator was developed in 1869 and such was the popularity of vibrators among women that they became the fifth household appliance to be electrified, beaten only by the sewing machine, fan, kettle and toaster!

When vibrators were portrayed as medical aids all was right with the world, but then pornographers began to depict their actual use. Censors frowned on these blatant acts of female sexuality and the vibrator was driven underground until work by sexologists, including Alfred Kinsey in the 1950s, brought female sexuality back into public discussion. And then, of course, we went through the swinging sixties, when sexuality became truly liberated and sex toys became ever more sophisticated, into the nineties when *Sex and the City* introduced us to the divine pleasures of the 'rabbit' perfectly constructed and perennially popular, mainstream and wholly acceptable to own.

Today's toys are more than simple playthings: they can improve vaginal muscle control and allow women who have never had an orgasm to experience one for the first time. Women often fall into two categories: those who would save their vibrator from their house if it were burning down and those who can't imagine what all the fuss is about. I want to take you through simple sex toys – and even those which sound more complicated or expensive often have cheaper versions for you to try out – so that you can learn to experiment with what takes your fancy, learn how to use them and find those that suit your needs and desires best. And while many of them are amazing used on your own, men are fascinated by them, how you use them and what you can do to him with them. So once you've mastered the art, bring them into your sex play with your partner too. Just remember that anything that penetrates needs to be used with a good water-based lubricant for ease of use and ultimate pleasure.

Why Use Sex Toys?

My immediate reply to my own question would be 'why not?' But they still remain a mystery for some people while others feel that they simply don't get the point of them. Perhaps I should start by debunking the top five myths about sex toys:

- **Sex toys are made for people who have sexual problems**
This myth probably originates from the days when sex toys were known as 'sex aids' or 'marital aids' and vibrators were prescribed to women as muscle relaxants and stress relievers. And while it's true that today's sex toys can help with these concerns – and more – they are designed for play, to enhance your sex life however amazing it is already.

- **Sex toys are there for people who don't have 'real' sex**
This particular myth is usually perpetrated by those that think of the kind of sex toys that sad, sexless and slightly weird men might want to use – blow-up dolls and the like. Failing to find a real partner, they have an imaginary, inflatable sexual 'friend'. Blow-up dolls are still out there, of course, but today's sex toys are used by men and women, both singles and couples.

- **If my partner uses a sex toy, she won't want sex with me any more . . .**
  Some men definitely feel threatened by vibrators and other sex toys. The ease with which a woman can have an orgasm makes them feel rather redundant. Guys, if you're thinking this – just don't go there. Vibrators are wonderful – but they are no real substitute for intimate, flesh-on-flesh, full-on foreplay and sex with your partner. And they're not great at taking us out for dinner, cuddling us through the night or putting out the rubbish either!

- **Sex toys are just for masturbation**
  Sex toy manufacturers are very careful not to market their products just for use when flying solo. And while they can be a great source of comfort, pleasure and expedience while masturbating, they can be just as much fun when shared with your partner.

- **Once I use a sex toy, I won't be able to get a normal orgasm**
  It's true that having an orgasm using a vibrator, or other sex toy, can be a lot faster and easier than having an orgasm through penetrative or oral sex. But using a sex toy will make absolutely no difference to your ability to have orgasms without one. You may have to be more patient and it may lack the intensity – or indeed be stronger – than an orgasm induced by a vibrator. You just have to learn to love the variety, that's all!

Vibrators

And so to the biggest market and most popular form of sex toy available. Why? Because they are by far the easiest way to have a clitoral orgasm. By stimulating the head of the clitoris in an intense, rhythmical way, it gives you a much easier, faster and more effective way to orgasm. Your partner's magic fingers or tongue might work wonders on your clitoris, but the truth is that the quickest and simplest route to an orgasm is via the vibrator. It may not be the most pleasurable sensation, in terms of that all-over fabulous orgasmic feeling that having sex with your lover brings, but hell, it's a fine alternative . . .

And although most vibrators come with a set of basic instructions, they tend to be functional rather than descriptive and a lot of women miss out on the real pleasure that a vibrator can bring, because they are just not sure how best to use it. A vibrator can be quite a shock to the system if you simply use them from cold, so you need to relax and do a little preparation beforehand.

Make sure that the room is warm and that you've gently felt around your vagina and clitoris to get you in the mood. You might like to watch a little porn while you're masturbating or listen to some sexy music or a song that makes you feel good. Always use some lubricant both on your vaginal opening and your clitoris as well as on the vibrator itself, where it will come into contact with your vagina. However much you may come to enjoy the intense top speed of your vibrator (and believe me, if you've never felt this, you're in for a treat!), always start revving up by using the lowest speed first. Start by applying a little pressure to your inner and outer labia, before moving the vibrator over your clitoral hood – the little piece of skin over the clitoris itself. It's a matter of trial and error – or how horny you're feeling – as to whether you'll want to apply direct, high-speed vibration to your clitoral hood or on to your clitoris. For some women, direct high vibration on the exposed clitoris can feel too intense. For others, it's a high-adrenalin rush to a dizzying orgasm. Just remember that there is no right or wrong way – just whatever feels right for you.

So what, among the vast array of shapes, colours, price points and promises are my own top recommendations? The best are available at lovehoney.co.uk or sextoys.co.uk.

- *The rabbit*

    This has to be top of the list, simply because it's the one women return to time and time again as the most enduringly satisfying vibrator on the market. It can be bought in many sizes – from a bullet-shaped handbag-size version to super size and at prices from £15 to over £100. There are rechargeable versions, rabbits with extra bead stimulation in the shaft, and names like Jessica, Jack and Mr Big, but what they all have in common – hence their name – is the little rabbit-ear attachment which vibrates at a rhythm to suit you, directly on your clitoris. Designed to be used along with the vibrating shaft, some women love their rabbit ears so much that they only use this part of the vibrator. Like any other sort of vibrator, it can be an expensive matter of trial and error to find the right one for you – as so much depends on your own pleasure and comfort zone in relationship to the size, mechanics and, in the case of the rabbit, the positioning and length of the rabbit ears in relationship to your clitoris. I suggest the **Rabbit Deluxe** or the **Jack Rabbit Pearl Vibrator** but my own personal can't-live-without favourite in performance terms, in spite of being a candy-coloured pink, is the **Slimline Passion Wave Jack Rabbit.** For luxury rabbits see pp. 143–45

- *Butterfly vibrators*

  Butterflies are vibrators specifically intended for clitoral stimulation. They are shaped like butterflies, with the main body concentrating the vibrations on the clitoris and the wings spreading additional vibrations around the genital region. Some of these can be strapped on, using a harness around your thighs. It's also hands free, so incredibly useful if you find operating the controls of a vibrator gives you tired arms! They cost between £10 and £50. My recommendation would be to go for the **Honeydew Butterfly** or for a bit of extra fun try the **OhMiBod Club Vibe Music Activated Vibrator.**

- *G-spot vibrators*

  You can also buy specially angled vibrators that are designed to maximise stimulation to your G-spot. They look much like any other vibrator, but tend to be longer than normal and have a curved end to make sure that you hit the spot. My recommendation would be to go for the **Slimline G-Spot Vibrator** or the **Vibrating Rock Chick G-Spot and Clitoral Vibrator.**

- *Bullet vibrators*

  These cheap little cuties are not much bigger than a lipstick, often made of metal or plastic and are very discreet – perfect as a travelling companion. They are designed to sit between the lips of the vagina and provide intense stimulation of your clitoris. They also work on your breasts, nipples and around the rim of your anus, providing a great buzz for you and your partner. There are some great ones made by **Candy Girl** and **Rock Chick**. For a real hit, try the **Colt Xtreme Turbo Bullet.**

- *Massagers*

  Not strictly marketed as sex toys at all, these are designed for stress release and relaxation. They deliver intense vibrations to the muscles that you can see, as well as those areas that are a little more discreetly tucked away on your body.

  There are a number of these on the market including the readily available **Philips Sensual Vibrating and Pulsating Massager.** The **Hitachi Magic Wand** has been America's favourite massage-style toy for a number of years and it's now available in the UK. Although it's a fairly unattractive product – it looks like a large old-fashioned microphone – it seems to hit the spot. One of the latest to hit the market – and getting rave reviews – is the **Eroscillator 2 Top Deluxe,** which provides amazing clitoral stimulation, but doesn't come in cheap at over £140. Bizarrely, it isn't rechargeable either – you'll need to use it while still plugged in, and on a very long cable, which makes it more cumbersome and less user-friendly than many other deluxe vibrators on the market.

Dildos

Dildos are named after the Italian term *diletta*, meaning delight, and have the general shape and appearance of a penis. This can range from highly realistic to vaguely penis-like. They also vary in colour, from rainbow to natural skin tones, and are made of rubber, latex, vinyl, plastic or jelly. There are also some rather beautiful ones around made of (toughened) glass that wouldn't look out of place on your window ledge or mantelpiece! They also vary enormously in size from the gently realistic to porn-star proportions. Although some dildos have built-in vibrators, the point is that they generally don't vibrate but are designed to either go in a strap-on harness or be used manually as a hard, penetrative stimulus. They are also known as dongs. They are best used while using a vibrator on your clitoris – as used on their own they can be a bit disappointing! The **Cyberskin Realistic Cock** is a good one to try, being pretty tough and realistic looking. Another alternative is the **Love Labs Ribbed Prober**. But the most important thing is that you find one that fits you well – they're like a perfect, customised penis – and getting the right shape and size is really important. Rather than spend a fortune finding out just what does suit you, try a 6- or 8-inch version – it usually does the trick.

Harnesses and Strap-ons

Harnesses are designed to hold a dildo or vibrator in place, usually for pleasuring another person. Some harnesses can hold both an external and an internal (or two internal) dildo or vibrator. It's actually a misconception that strap-ons are devices solely for lesbians; in fact they are used far more often by heterosexual women performing anal sex on their partner. Lots of men love the feeling of having a toy that's connected to their partner's body thrusting in and out of them, while for women, strap-on sex is a new way to give their partner pleasure. Harnesses can be made of leather, vinyl, nylon or rubber and can be hugely expensive. Some women just find them too uncomfortable to wear (and heavy dildos just have a habit of falling out!) but if you fancy trying one, the **Vivid Designer Harness** range is worth a look. The **Wireless Latex Harness with Slender Penis** is also good, if you find some of the dildos just look too big! The most important thing is to find one that fits securely and comfortably. Given that you are likely to be buying your harness online, this can prove a difficult choice to make, so try and go for one that is adjustable and has as many straps and buckles as possible.

Cock Rings

The main reason cock rings were developed was in order to keep blood in the penis to make a guy have a longer and harder erection. But many have been developed that have little 'nubs', sometimes vibrating, on the end so that a woman can get clitoral stimulation at the same time. And they really can make a difference to your clitoral pleasure when having sex. When your lover wears one, make sure that the little vibrating nub is on the top of his penis, so that it not only stimulates the base of his penis but also gives you maximum clitoral stimulation. They work best when you're in the missionary position, or when there is fairly close and frequent penetrative contact, otherwise too much full in-and-out thrusting can mean that the nub isn't really doing its work! The good news is that cock rings are pretty cheap and fairly disposable. There's a huge variety costing from a couple of quid upwards. **Screaming O** makes a good range and the elegantly designed **Lelo BO** is rechargeable.

Butt Plugs

Butt plugs are toys designed to be inserted into the anus. They can be simple A-shaped devices, realistically moulded penises, or exotic shapes. They feature a flange (a flared device) on one end so that they don't slide inside the body and are available in a variety of materials including plastics, rubber and jelly. They must be used with a really good lubricant and are great for experimenting with, especially if this is your first time to anal sex. As they are designed to go into your bottom and stay there, they leave your hands to do other stuff while they open up your rectum. Men especially enjoy butt plugs as they reach to the male G-spot – the prostate gland. **Doc Johnson** has a wide range of butt plugs at all prices.

Anal Beads

Like butt plugs, anal beads must be used with copious amounts of lubricants. They give you the ability to enjoy one particular sensation several times over – when your sphincter muscles relax, the anus opens up, a bead slides in and the muscles close around it. While most anal bead toys have between five and ten separate beads, make sure that you buy a good quality set made of one continuous piece of rubber or silicone. The problem with some of the cheaper models is that they are made of hard plastic beads on a piece of nylon or cotton string – not only impossible to clean and disinfect but also unsafe as the beads have rough edges and might even come off during playtime, which is absolutely not what you want, unless a trip to A & E is part of your playtime fun! Try **Mantric Dinky Vibrating Anal Beads** or a set made by **Booty Beads.**

Clitoral Stimulators

Clitoral stimulators are designed to directly stimulate the clitoris and while they usually vibrate, there are also non-powered clitoral stimulators that work by rubbing against the clitoris when walking or moving around. While many women report good results from these, others simply find then intrusive or uncomfortable – neither feelings are conducive to having an orgasm! Clitoral stimulators come in both strap-on and hand-held varieties. The two most popular clitoral stimulators are the rabbits and the butterflies. If you want to try a vibrator designed especially for clitoral stimulation, either just use the ears of your rabbit, **Jimmyjane's FORM 2** (see p. 144) or try the **Waterproof Clitoral Hummer** designed for women, by women!

Luxury Sex Toys

There are a whole host of luxury sex toys out there on the market. And by luxury, I don't just mean seriously expensive – some of the platinum versions cost up to £4000 – but rather beautiful, designer-inspired, amazing objects in their own right. The thing about luxury toys is that the more expensive they become, the less they look like what they are meant to do. Very few look like a penis – most are slightly alien-like, or look like a cigar case, pebble or a mobile phone. Some are designed, in fact, to work with your mobile phone or your MP3 player. And many are, sadly, a triumph of form over function. However, a number of them have been developed clinically, using the most advanced technology available, manufactured using medical-grade silicone in beautiful jewel-like colours, and amazingly work just as they should: delivering first-class orgasms. At a first-class price, of course. But they should also deliver a lifetime's worth of pleasure – which makes them worth every penny.

None of my special favourites will leave you much change from £100, but all these are guaranteed to deliver amazing service and somehow, because they are intrinsically beautiful objects in themselves, there is something very special about using them that adds to your pleasure. For my money, buying just one of these will serve you well. They tend to be waterproof, discreet and rechargeable and added to your favourite, penis-shaped vibrator, you will have an orgasmic repertoire on your hands for every mood. And if these seem too much of an investment for you, remember that these are currently state-of-the-art vibrators and there will always be something similar – and much cheaper – available if you do a bit of shopping around.

They tend to fall into four categories: rabbit-type vibrators, lay-ons (non-penetrative vibrators), classic vibrators and massagers. Depending on your preferences, these are my front-runners for a luxury vibrator. That's not to say that there aren't others around, but based on pretty extensive (and pleasurable) research these items win hands down for combining style, quality, low noise levels and functionality – that is, delivering that orgasm as often as you like . . .

Rabbits

In an ever-crowded market, manufacturers have become aware, through extensive market analysis, that the shaft of the rabbit-style vibrator is only really needed as a handle to manoeuvre the ears into position over and around our clitoris! So with this in mind, my leading contender in this category really just consists of some very sophisticated rabbit ears indeed!

Jimmyjane FORM 2 Waterproof Rechargeable Vibrator
FORM 2 combines all the orgasmic fun of the buzzing ears of a rabbit vibrator with the kind of intensity normally reserved for mains-powered sex toys! Small, petite and beautiful, this multi-function Jimmyjane vibrator is part of the groundbreaking 'Pleasure to the People' series – a gorgeous collection of waterproof, rechargeable vibrators that seamlessly mix incomparable power with creative design.

Made from silicone, with unique shaping – it looks a bit like a mini Space Hopper – the FORM 2 uses the tried, tested and adored 'rabbit ears' design and combines it with two synchronised vibrators that are located in the very tips of the sex toy.

Easy to use and pleasing to hold against the body, FORM 2 features three simple buttons that control the intensity, speed and function of vibration, as well as turning it on and off. It's also very quiet, and its small and discreet shape means that you can take it anywhere, making it the perfect travel companion! Jimmyjane have taken a simple idea, reinvented it and managed to revolutionise the clitoral orgasm!

Lelo Ina Luxury Rechargeable Rabbit Vibrator
A really beautifully designed, ergonomically pleasing vibrator that gives a new and rather sophisticated twist on the classic rabbit vibrator design and shape. While the curved shaft is designed to target the G-spot, the 'rabbit' ear is much firmer than on most vibrators and so delivers quite an intense sensation on to your clitoris. Not only does it have the variable speeds and modes that you'd expect from a vibrator of this quality, it has an amazing device that, by the way of two individual vibrating motors, manages to allow one sensual area to heighten in intensity while the vibration level can be lowered on the other part. Another product made from silicone, it's smart, sexy and so quiet as to be almost silent – which are what Lelo toys are all about.

Lay-ons

Some women find the intensity of a clitoral vibrator just too much, especially if they have a sensitive clitoris, and these non-penetrative vibrators, known as 'lay-ons' – for pretty obvious reasons – provide the perfect, more gentle alternative.

SaSi by Je Joue Intelligent Rechargeable Vibrator

This is shaped like a large, very pretty, double pebble with a ball bearing underneath its oh-so-soft silicone skin. It vibrates against your vulva and the little ball bearing is the closest that any toy, in my view, has come to simulating oral sex. Its smooth massaging ball circles under a soft silicone skin, while vibrating and pulsating to create unique caresses and sheet-clenching stimulation. And SaSi learns what you like while you use it, so every time you switch on, you're guaranteed your favourite turn-on. There are two modes – favourite, which goes through all the functions, and customised, which you can adapt to your own needs and it remembers what you like as well as having a handy 'don't stop' button. SaSi comes pre-loaded with what Je Joue calls 'Sensual Intelligence', which customises the orgasm experience just for you. It learns what you like and what you don't like – and then remembers this for future pleasure. Not to mention that it's splash-proof, quiet and so discreet that it's easy to take with you when you're on your travels.

What is so amazing – and unique – about this fabulous little toy is its combination of gentle vibration and movement that manages to deliver a really sensational, slower and more sensual form of orgasm than most other vibrators.

Lelo Lily Luxury Rechargeable Vibrator

In keeping with many products in the Lelo range – and not dissimilar to the slightly cheaper **Nea** – the smooth and silky pearl-like surface of the Lily, made out of a smooth coated plastic, both feels and looks beautiful and its multiple speeds are designed to give you vibrations all the way from a slow, gentle buzz right up to truly intense vibrations. Another travel-friendly item, once again it's quiet and discreet.

Classic vibrators

Once upon a time, before the sex-toy market got all sophisticated, high-tech and competitive, all vibrators could have been considered 'classic'. Without any whistles, bells, patterns and modes, they were simply phallic-shaped objects, designed for inserting into the vagina for a vaginal orgasm. They seemed to 'eat' batteries – there's little more frustrating than having to find replacement batteries in the middle of your self-pleasure – and were incredibly noisy: there was nothing discreet about using one of these! Now, thankfully, a new generation of classic luxury vibrators has arrived with beautiful designs, gentle curving shapes, all manner of vibration speeds and modes and, as they're rechargeable, you'll never have to worry about spent batteries again.

Jimmyjane FORM 6 Luxury Rechargeable Massager

A powerhouse of a product, the FORM 6 with its multiple speeds provides amazing digital vibrations ranging from gentle oscillations to exhilarating pulses, yet with all this power still manages to be virtually silent. It is a toy to be used as you wish – the continuous contours made from silicone mean that there is no specific end that you hold on to or apply to your body. In fact, I think it works much better as an external vibrator, rather than a penetrative one. But if you do insert the smaller end inside your vagina, the outer part sits very comfortably against your vulva and clitoris.

G-Ki by Je Joue Adjustable G-Spot Vibrator

The rechargeable G-Ki is one of the first G-spot toys to take into consideration the fact that not everyone is built the same. It's made of silicone and is bendable so that it can be shaped to fit your body, giving you perfect and precise access to your G-spot as well as giving you simultaneous clitoral stimulation.

At the top of the G-Ki, you'll find a special button (the one with three dots) that can be pressed in, allowing you to adjust the angle of this G-spot-seeking head. Once you've found your G-spot and the head is in the perfect location, you can then use the button further down the shaft (the one with five dots) to curve the body of the G-Ki around and rest it against your clitoris and labia.

As well as being adjustable, the G-Ki also manages to feature five powerful speeds and five different vibration pulses in both the G-spot and the clitoral part of the toy. It's also quiet and submersible in water.

Lelo Elise Luxury Rechargeable Vibrator
With five intense pleasure modes and virtually silent in its performance, the Elise is a clitoral and G-spot vibrator in one.

Like so many of these luxury vibrators, its beauty lies in its simplicity. It's tactile, gorgeous to look at and provides hours of bliss with its 'twin engined' pleasure points and five simulation modes. The Elise will even indicate when it's time to recharge, so you need never get caught out mid-flow!

Massagers

Philips Sensual Dual Intimate Massagers
There are very few sex toys out there that are designed to be used by couples. Most of them are pretty much

exclusively male or female and designed to be used from a woman to a man and vice versa.

Philips, however, has developed a range of toys for couples – rather coyly called 'massagers' – and the flagship product in this range is the Sensual Dual Intimate Massagers. This set of two luxury vibrating massagers made from rubber allows you to explore each other slowly and their non-phallic design makes them ideal for newcomers to the world of sex toys. They're also quiet, which is a bonus. The massager designed to be used on women is long with a rounded, almost bulbous, tip, whereas the male massager is smooth and contoured, ideal for using on the perineum and testicles. Both have variable settings so that you can control the speed.

The massagers are splash-proof and recharge in their own specially designed discreet case.

Nomi Tang Better Than Chocolate Multi-Function Clitoral Massager Vibrator

Another excellent non-penetrative vibrator is the fabulously named 'Better Than Chocolate', made by Nomi Tang. Beautifully packaged and designed, this lovely little vibrator is ergonomically and sensually shaped but definitely packs a clitoral punch. Made of rubber, it can be submerged into water to give you some bathtime thrills.

Easy and quiet to use, it has a touch-sensitive, light-up bar to control the range of pulsation to suit you.

A Final Word on Safety . . .

While an STI (Sexually Transmitted Infection) doesn't tend to live long outside the body, it is rare but possible to catch one from a sex toy. Although they are inanimate objects, they might well come into contact with all sorts of bodily fluids – semen, vaginal fluids, rectal bacteria and so on. So it is absolutely essential to keep your toys as clean as possible.

Some toys, especially those designed to be inserted into the anus, should be sterilised if possible, while most non-penetrative toys can simply be cleaned with a wet wipe. Not all toys are waterproof – or even splash-proof – so check the instructions before you go plunging them into a basin of warm soapy water.

4 Sex Games: Games, Kits and DIY

This book has been all about sex games – whether that's fantasies, role play or sex toys. But what about games, pure and simple? (Okay, maybe not so pure or simple, but you know what I mean.) Those games you can buy online or from Ann Summers – neatly packaged and colourfully boxed up, offering hours of unabated pleasure. They usually contain some combination of an ostrich feather, furry handcuffs or binding material, a blindfold and some suggestive cards.

As games go many of them don't offer great value for money and are a bit 'samey'. The quality of them tends to vary – but even the most expensive will have poor-quality props and most of them are simply a not very imaginative variation of the others. Unlike the world of extraordinarily well-developed and advanced sex toys, boxed games themselves are generally not nearly as sophisticated in their presentation or function and there are very few of them on the market so they end up being a bit tacky and predictable. However, the suggestion or question cards can be fun, erotic and give you all sorts of ideas to spice up your sex life. My advice to you would be to invest in the better of the ready-made games, buy your own props, abandon the rules of the game and simply keep the cards to use in many of the 'home-made' game suggestions that I describe later on in this chapter.

Here are the three best games out there – what you get for your money and how you play them. My team of willing researchers and I have tried and tested most of the games around, and these three were found to be way ahead of the competition.

Boxed Games

Nookii – the grown-up game for playful couples
Priced around £25

Contents:
90 Nookii cards
Timer
Two dice
Sheer scarf

'Do Not Disturb' sign
Directions for the game

This is one of the best pre-packaged games around. Rather than move around a playing board, you move around each other's body, following the suggestions on the 'Mmm', 'Ooh' and 'Aah' cards. There are different cards designed for men and women.

Basically, the 'Mmm' cards are a gentle warm-up to get you in the mood, the 'Ooh' cards are fun-based role play so you can go a little further and the 'Aah' cards are more advanced and 'naughty'.

Examples of the cards include:

Mmm cards

For a woman
- *Lie down on your side with your head resting on your hand.*

  'Lie down behind me on your side. Slip your hands under my top and playfully cover my chest with delicate figures of eight. Lick your fingers and start to give my nipples attention by tweaking and employing gentle circular movements.

  'Move downwards and spend some time applying a figure of eight on my stomach area. Move your hands down further, teasing my inner thighs.'

For a man
- *Sit in a chair.*

'Run your fingers through my hair, pulling it gently away from my ears. Gently kiss my neck and rub the outer edges of one ear with your thumb and fore-finger, moving up and down several times.

'Plant delicate kisses all around the outline of my ear and nibble me lightly with your lips. Suck my earlobe, saturating it completely. Blow your breath so I feel it hard and hot in the centre. Probe me with your tongue.'

Ooh cards
For a woman
- *Wear just your bra and panties.*

'Lay me on my tummy and kneel down beside me. Stroke the back of my thighs, slowly working up to my bum.'

Raise your bottom in the air.

'Run your nails lightly over my buttocks. Massage my bum with your fingertips, gently at first but drifting into firm squeezing and kneading. Pull my cheeks apart slightly and apply little nibbles and soft kisses.'

Wiggle your bottom rhythmically in synch with the attention it's receiving.

For a man

- *Strip down to your underpants.*

'Pull my pants up high between my cheeks like a thong, exposing my buttocks. Order me on all fours. Apply rapid kisses to my feet, moving upwards to cover my body; along my thighs, my half-bared bottom, my naked back and my neck.

'When you reach my head ask me to lie on my back. Ease the pace of your pecking to bite my nipples and kiss my chest.'

Aah cards

For a woman

- *Strip naked and lean back against a wall with your legs open.*

'Get on your knees and kiss my feet. Lick the inside of my legs and kiss my knees.'
Clasp your lover's head.

'Lick the inside of my thighs, taking time to teasingly nibble the fleshy parts.'
Part your legs further and guide your lover's head between your legs.

'Lick me lovingly.'

For a man

- *Strip totally naked and kneel down in front of my face with your knees together.*

'Place both hands upon my head. Run your fingers through my hair. Part your knees and cover your top with the scarf and bring yourself towards my face. Clasp my scalp and using all your fingers in a circular motion, massage me. Lightly scratch down my back, underneath my panties and across my cheeks. Rock yourself rhythmically against my face.'

(Cards reproduced by kind permission of www.nookii.com)

The cards are fun and suggestive and the beauty of this game is that you can move progressively through the three stages of the game, making the journey feel more like foreplay, rather than a random order of events. It also feels like the instructions on the cards have actually been written by a real person with a sensitive under-standing of sexual fun, rather than the robotic and slightly ridiculous suggestions used by other games of poorer quality. In their own words, 'Nookii is a map of foreplay, a key to a door of possibilities on a multitude of sensual interactions.'

Monogamy – a hot affair with your partner
Priced around £25

Contents:
Playing board
100 cards for him, featuring 300 questions at three levels
100 cards for her, featuring 300 questions at three levels
50 fantasy cards
Dice, two player's pieces and twelve level pieces
Set of easy reference rules

Like Nookii, Monogamy – one of the earliest and best games on the market – works well because it's a progressive game, with the questions becoming more intimate and the challenges more exciting as you move around the board. The three levels of cards begin with 'Intimate' questions, move on to 'Passionate' questions and then to the final 'Steamy' level. The game concludes with the winner choosing one of the 50 fantasy cards to play out for real. Developed by a delightful, real-life couple who wanted to spice up their own sex life, Monogamy is one of the best games of its kind and even has a fan club of people who say that it has genuinely turned their sex lives around!

Examples of the cards include:

Intimate

Hers

'Your brief is to plan a weekend for your partner, with no expense spared, which would blow his mind. Let him know what he could look forward to.'

His

'Do you prefer the lights on or off when you are making love? Well, don't keep her in the dark... Explain.'

Hers

'Ask your partner to tell you something about himself that perhaps you are unaware of. Now return the compliment.'

His

'Getting In A Lather. Why is a shaved pubis an object of desire for many men? And are women who shave turned on by it? Welcome to the cutting edge of sexual debate.'

Passionate

Hers

'Acquired Taste. Can you think of a sexual activity that once switched you off and now turns you on? What was it that pressed the right button?'

His
'Suspense! Has your partner any suspenders hidden away in her lingerie drawer? If so, ask her to put them on now and keep them on for the rest of the game if you both so wish.'

Hers
'Taste Test. Blindfold your partner and go to the kitchen. Choose three things that you can dip your fingers into and let your partner suck them off. Can he guess what they are? If you're feeling really naughty swap one of the liquids for some honey from your love cup!'

His
'Toy Department. There are countless sex toys on the market nowadays, particularly for women. Ask which would give her the most pleasure. Perhaps you may have a suggestion or two!'

Steamy
Hers
'Check Your Writing. Ancient oriental texts suggest that a woman's upper mouth lip is directly connected to her clitoris. Get him to test your circuitry by simultaneously nibbling your top lip and caressing your clitoris. Warning: you may blow a fuse!'

His

'Feel The Lash Of Her Tongue. As a punishment (for nothing in particular) you are going to be tied to a chair, brought to full erection by your partner and then whipped into a frenzy of excitement by her tongue flicking rapidly over your helmet for two delicious minutes. You deserve everything you get.'

Hers

'Puss In Boots. Wearing your sexiest high heels or boots – and nothing else – give him a two-minute floor show, with Puss in the spotlight. Make sure he gets a front-row view, but if he tries to touch you, the show's over!'

His

'Recognise The Taste? Ask her to sit on your face and really smear her juices all over. After a few minutes, while your face is still moist, give her a deep French kiss. Does she like a taste of her own medicine?'

Fantasy

'Good Clean Fun.

'Showers could well have been made as a sex toy. They combine heat, moisture, pressure and friction all in one handy little innocent-looking device. So why not get yours working for the two of you. Hop in the shower with generous lashings of sensuous shower gel and start by covering each other in lather. Use the jets of water from the showerhead to masturbate each other and to clean all those hard to reach places! The best position for shower sex is definitely for her to bend over while he penetrates her from behind, so go on, get down to some good clean fun! (Silicone lubricant that stays on even in water is great to make sure he slips in rather than slips over.)'

'Ripping Yarn.

'It only ever seems to happen in the movies, but now it can happen in the comfort and privacy of your own home! Yes, this is your chance to experience the sounds and the sensations of ripping each other's clothes off in a passionate frenzy, literally ripping, as in tearing. So, both put on some old clothes that you don't mind consigning to the bin (tights especially lend themselves to this game). One of you goes and hides somewhere, while the other acts as a hunter. You both know what the hunter is after and the chase merely heightens the level of lust on both sides. Once the quarry is found, there is a mad, mutual outpouring of passion, accompanied by the sound of material being ripped to shreds, heavy breathing and whirlwind orgasms.'

(Cards reproduced by kind permission of
www.creativeconceptions.com)

Risky or Frisky? – a hot affair with your partner
Priced around £25

Contents:
Playing board
100 risky or frisky cards
100 question cards
25 business cards
2 dice
8 playing pieces
Risky or Frisky? currency notes
Rule sheet

Unlike Nookii or Monogamy, Risky or Frisky? is designed to be played not only as a couple, but also with what they describe as 'friends and very good friends' – the aim of the game is to build the most successful adult business. And indeed they would have to be pretty good friends as some of the action on the way to winning can get very steamy indeed. Even the playing pieces are shaped like mini rabbit vibrators for her and mini cock rings for him!

Examples of the cards include:

Risky
You have won first prize in a cross-dressing competition. Collect 100 notes from each player!

Your car is clamped whilst visiting the local strip club. Pay 200 notes for its release!

Frisky
Change clothes with another player. If you do it within 60 secs, each collect 250 notes. Keep your undies to yourself for this task!

It's a full moon: are you a vampire or a wolf? Either way your teeth will be razor sharp. Nibble a player's neck and body for one minute. If they laugh collect 100 notes and if they moan with joy collect 250 notes.

Question cards
Q: What does BDSM stand for?
A: Bondage, Discipline, Sadism and Masochism

Q: What % of men admit to masturbating at least once a day?
A: 54%

Q: The sexual act of rubbing to achieve sexual pleasure without penetration is more commonly known as what?
A: Frottage

Business cards

Strip Club/Adult Dating Website/DVD Distributor, etc.

These cards represent the rent you can charge if you own one or more of a similar company.

(Cards reproduced by kind permission of
www.riskyorfrisky.com)

What makes these high-quality games stand out in a fairly impoverished market is that they build up your sexual anticipation in a realistic way as well as offering suggestions, information, questions and challenges that can't fail to fire up your sex life. These and other similar games are readily available from sex toy sites such as sextoys.co.uk and lovehoney.co.uk.

Kits

There are also some wonderful kits out there on the market. They are so beautifully packaged that simply opening them up and investigating the contents is a pleasure in itself.

Bijoux Indiscrets make some lovely and unusual games, all packaged in highly covetable black 'lace' tins that would make a gorgeous gift for your partner.

Though they sound very sexy and French, they are in fact made in Spain and are available online in specialist outlets. The best include:

Poême: includes an inkpot full of chocolate sauce, a satin mask and a feather quill pen flume for writing in chocolate on your lover's body.

L'eau à Deux: a bath kit that includes massage oil, sensual bath foam, a music CD, scented candles and a massager.

Agent Secret: a James Bond-type game in a tin that includes soft tying-up ribbons, a feather tickler, a mask, lock and a secret mission card.

Coffret Bling Bling: a sexy role-play game that includes shiny body powder, a feather tickler and furry handcuffs.

Regard Indiscret: a role-play game that includes high-quality nipple covers, a pearl belt, scented candles and a soft feather boa.

The clever people at the House of Nookii also make their own kits – the packaging and contents are a little less sophisticated than the Bijoux Indiscrets range, but nevertheless they are fun, playful and a great way to fire up your imagination, sex-game wise. Their products all contain a little vibrator and massager as well as accessories like role-play cards and blindfolds.

Check out their fun website, www.nookii.com, for more details on these kits:

In the Mood for Love
Ooh La La Rabbit Kit
Slap & Tickle for Couples
Weekend Fun Collection

Jimmyjane also make an adorable and beautifully packaged little kit, called *Indulgences* that includes a black feather tickler, mini bullet vibrator, a packet of condoms, sachets of lubricant and a little game in itself, called a love decoder. It would make a fabulous gift.

Your Sex-game Toy Box

But what if you want to build your own customised game – something where you get to choose your own props and your own questions and fantasies? Firstly you'll need a basic wardrobe of props and accessories. I suggest the following, which all have the added bonus of being able to be used during the fantasies and role play recommended elsewhere in this book:

Pillows

This sounds like a basic prerequisite for having sex but having a good and plentiful supply of comfortable pillows and cushions can make a huge difference to your sex games as they can be used for propping yourself up in all sorts of positions, ensuring that your hands, knees and elbows avoid carpet burns or the distracting and unwanted pain that a hard wooden floor can bring.

A timer

A number of games are more exciting when there is a time restriction on them, so use a kitchen or an egg timer, or a stopwatch, to keep the momentum going.

A blindfold

You can use virtually anything for this: a silky scarf, a stocking, a man's necktie, an airline sleeping mask or a blindfold specially designed for sex purposes. Blindfolds add to the fun because they work on sensory deprivation. Not being able to see what is happening to you adds to the intensity of your feelings. Wearing a blindfold means that each lick, nibble and stroke is full of sensory surprise. You can buy leather, silk or sequinned blindfolds or just use a traditional scarf – you don't need fancy equipment for this sensation.

Restraints

Designed for the ankles or the wrists, these can be handcuffs (furry and gentle or steel and severe!), bondage tape or a silk scarf or stocking. Handcuffs or arm restraints are essential in bondage play. Most handcuffs are made of leather or leather-look plastic, but depending on your preference you can go for the heavy-duty police variety (just don't lose the key!) or the furry, fun variety. You can also use special bondage tape or simply a silk or cotton scarf – anything that will keep your partner from moving their arms or hands, but won't actually stop their circulation altogether!

Paddles, whips and riding crops

Whips and paddles are designed to help you and your partner straddle that pain–pleasure divide with varying degrees. Using whips and spanking paddles is a harmless and provocative way of spicing up your sex life and opening up new sexual avenues for you and your partner to explore. Indulge yourself and your partner in some punishment role play by using a whip or spanking paddle to dish out small amounts of pain in response to naughty activities. No paddle? Use a hairbrush handle or a wooden spoon instead.

Although crops can leave you feeling fabulously in control, they do deliver a more intense, localised sensation than a paddle. A whip can be even more unruly as the tails can have a wraparound effect, catching vulnerable parts of the body, like the hips and kidneys, so unless you're an expert at using one of these, keep to one with short and lightweight strands.

Harnesses and strap-ons

Not essential in playing games at all, unless you're going for something quite racy, but they are an interesting addition to the sexual toy box. Harnesses are designed to hold a dildo or vibrator in place, usually for pleasuring another person. Some harnesses can hold both an external and an internal (or two internal) dildo or vibrator. There's more on harnesses and strap-ons on p. 138.

An ostrich feather

Gentle and sensuous, the soft plumes of an ostrich feather are best for sex play. Used with a blindfold so that the sense of touch becomes even more acute, the effects can be quite overwhelming, in the sexiest possible way.

A silk scarf

One of the most adaptable and versatile props you can use – it can be used as a blindfold, a restraint, a veil or a sensual, stroking accessory. You can even use it as a mouth gag.

Massage oil

Whether you're using baby oil or a specialist, scented massage oil, the extra glide that oils can provide can make a big difference in sex play.

Scented candles

An essential in many sex games. Not only do scented candles give off an ambient and very sexy lighting effect and smell gorgeous, they also shed a very forgiving light for those who lack confidence in their own bodies or are inexperienced in sex games. Use them to vary the atmosphere – musky, pungent smells when you're playing something rough and naughty and flowery, more gentle scents when you're in a more romantic mood.

Remember that all these items are just the basics for play and you can add to these as your enthusiasm and experience grows. Some of them can be incredibly beautiful – and frighteningly expensive – so start off with the cheaper models until you've worked out what works best for you and your partner.

Before I move on to some ideas for other games you can play, let's look at just a few of the more unusual items you can use to enhance your sex games. Remember that there are many others – you are only as limited as far as your imagination and your store cupboard/freezer/wardrobe will let you go . . .

Ice

Remember that delicious sensation of an ice cube melting on your body on a really hot day? Amazingly cool relief from the sun; a slightly shocking feeling that actually it was way too cold. That sensation is a fairly mild form of pain–pleasure syndrome, so beloved of BDSM (Bondage, Domination, Submission and Masochism) enthusiasts, but playing with ice doesn't need to travel into very extreme situations and can be fun.

When things steam up in the bedroom or you're in a secluded but public place, take a small ice cube and gently use your finger to trace a pattern over your partner's body. Glide the ice across their nipples, down towards their tummy and then tease a little between their thighs. If you're a little more secluded, take the ice cube in your mouth and do the same thing. Let your tongue lap away the droplets formed by the melting ice.

Men: You can also use an ice cube to numb up your lover's labia, which gives an amazing feeling especially if aroused.

Women: If your man can bear it, and the sensation is not too acute, you can also use a slightly melted ice cube to stroke over his perineum and anal opening. If all this seems just too frosty, simply sucking an ice cube also makes your mouth lovely and cold when you give your partner oral sex.

You can also use those fruit-flavoured ice pops to trace around your partner's inner arms, backs of knees and inner thighs – those places where the skin is thinnest and most sensitive.

Wax

Like ice play, wax play has that naughty but nice element, only it has the added bonus of being slightly dangerous – so do take care when using melted candles. Plain white candles are the best for wax games as they burn at the lowest temperature, while beeswax candles are definitely to be avoided – they can cause severe burning. If in doubt, test a few drops of wax on your own skin before trying it out on your partner. Some of the sex toy companies also produce special massage candles, which burn at low temperatures, and are designed for wax play. The Jimmyjane range of massage candles are fairly expensive but they are really quite special and a little goes a long, long way . . .

So what do you do with this sort of pain play? You could try blindfolding your partner and letting some drops of wax fall on random parts of their body. It's best to keep to the tummy or back and avoid the genitals at all costs – this is most definitely not an area for wax play!

While you may enjoy playing out this fantasy, your partner may hate it, so proceed with caution both in safety and sympathetic terms – peeling it away from the skin can also produce an intense sensation that some couples like.

Desk fan

Positioning a small desk fan near you while you play sex games can be really stimulating. The cool stream of low-speed air against your or your partner's genitals and backside provides a shivery and teasing sensation that adds pleasure to the more intimate games that you play.

Stockings

Yes, of course *wearing* stockings can be a big part of sex games, but if you're a woman, try wearing them on your hands like a pair of gloves – the silkier and more sheer the better. You can use them to give your partner a sensual massage over his body or his penis.

Hair scrunchie

A fabric ponytail holder or two can be a great addition to playing sex games. You can use it as a hand or ankle restraint or wrap it, not too tightly, around your partner's penis, to provide the sort of pressure that is exciting without being too painful.

Cotton wool balls

Soaking cotton wool balls in a sweet liqueur like Baileys or Malibu and running it along your partner's penis, testicles and anus and licking it as you go can be a – literally – delicious game. The alcohol also evaporates quickly, leaving a tingling cool sensation on those especially sensitive areas, rich in nerve endings.

MASSAGE

Massage is not a sex game in itself, but it can be incorporated into role play or just become part of your normal repertoire. Don't worry if you're not experienced in the art of massage – by being sensitive to your partner's oral or visual cues, you'll soon discover if what you are imparting is pleasurable or otherwise!

Set aside an hour for the ultimate in sensual massage, and make sure that any distractions – mobile phones in particular – are switched off! Think of the massage as three separate sections: the beginning, when you make your partner as relaxed, responsive and receptive as possible, the middle, when your massage becomes sexy and teasing, and the last twenty minutes, when you will give your partner the ultimate genital massage.

To begin:

Setting the scene

- turn the lights down low or light candles
- make the room as quiet as possible or play soft, soothing music
- ensure you have the right massage oil to hand. Use only a few drops of essential oils to a plain base as too much can smell overwhelming and can burn skin.

The massage

- get your partner to lie face down on some soft towels
- warm the massage oil in your hands
- run your oiled fingertips down the length of your lover's back
- once they are relaxed, use firmer strokes and a little more pressure
- move your hands in mirroring movements, using firm circular motions in and away from the backbone
- work your way down their back, paying special attention to their shoulders
- when you reach the small of the back, use just your palms, pushing them firmly into the small of the back and work your way down to the buttocks and then back up again

The middle:

- turn your partner over and start massaging their chest or breasts, working from the top to the bottom
- women's breasts can be sensitive or painful before or during her period so be gentle
- be guided by your partner's verbal responses to what you're doing
- make the next twenty minutes as sexy and as teasing as possible, building up anticipation for . . .

Genital massage – the ultimate hand job:

Male genital massage

- bend or kneel down so that you are between your man's legs
- gently roll your fingers and thumb over his testicles
- cup his testicles in your palms and use your fingers to stroke the ultra-sensitive skin of his scrotal sacs
- hold the base of his penis firmly with one hand while using the other to spiral and twist up the shaft of his penis to the head
- as his erection stiffens, use the palm and open fingers of your hand to rub back and forth over the head of his penis

- the tip of his penis should be a little wet, but you can use some lubricant to make the sensation even more pleasurable for him
- you can bring a man to orgasm in this way, or you may want to have penetrative sex at this point, but make sure that you don't suddenly decrease the pressure, as this can be frustrating for him

Female genital massage

- Use an unscented, water-based lubricant as the vagina is too sensitive for perfumed products
- kneel between her open legs, and use your palm and fingertips to brush along her inner thighs, creating different levels of pressure as you do so
- tease and lightly touch her genitals, and rhythmically caress her tummy, breasts and nipples
- when you determine your partner is ready, in a circular motion gently tease the outer labia, or lips, of her vagina. You should be able to tell how turned on she is feeling through her sighs of pleasure, or from visual clues – her labia may begin to glisten and start to deepen in colour

- now's the time to touch her clitoris – roll your finger gently over or around it but do not squeeze or pinch as this is the most sensitive part of a woman's vagina
- if this is making her feel good gradually increase the pressure as you circle her clitoris; if it seems too sensitive, go back to touching her labia
- her breathing and moans should tell you that she's approaching orgasm. Using more lubrication if necessary, gently push a finger or two into her vagina, continuing to pay attention to her clitoris
- if you turn your fingertips upwards, you may be able to feel her G-spot, a raised area with a slightly ridged texture. Use a firm but gentle beckoning gesture as if you're pulling her towards you from within
- continue in this way, bringing your partner to orgasm

Let the Games Begin . . .

Whether you buy a ready-made board game complete with props or decide to customise or invent your own, these are some of the simpler games that will really fire up your juices.

Keeping Control

The control in this game is all about controlling your orgasm. Other than penetrative sex, do whatever it takes to bring your partner to orgasm. Oral sex, a hand job, kissing or licking their erogenous zones. Spend around half a minute or so doing this and then swap places and let your partner choose to do something to you. You can even try the 69 position where you're performing oral sex on each other. The object of the game is to get your partner to have an orgasm before you, though to be honest there are no 'losers' in this game, which will probably break all the rules after a while . . .

Secret Desires

This game is all about those desires that you'd like to find out about your partner – given a certain situation, what would he or she really like to do to or with you? Make up 30 cards or so – you can use suggestions from existing board games or create your own ideas – and then get your partner to pick a card and fill in the blanks. Examples for your cards could include:

'The most sexy surprise you could give me would be to _____'

'I wish we did more _____ in bed'

'You could really turn me on by _____'

'I really love it when you kiss my _____'

'If we were alone for the night and you could play with one sexy prop with me, it would be a _____'

Easy As ABC

This is just a simple little game where you get your partner to start with the letter 'A' and he or she has to kiss an area of your body beginning with that letter. Then you have to do the same for a body part beginning with the letter 'B' and so on. It's clearly much easier for some letters than others – but this is where your imagination, inventiveness (and knowledge of sexual slang!) comes into play.

Pantie Play

The trick of this game is to remove your partner's pants, using only your mouth and teeth – no hands are allowed. Whether you wear briefs or a thong is entirely up to you – and you might want to try some of those knickers made of edible candy that you can buy at Ann Summers or online.

Just A Minute

No, not the Radio 4 panel game (though that could be interesting too, if you just allow yourselves to talk about sexual positions, fantasies or erogenous zones!) but an opportunity to take turns to choose one area of your partner's body, and spend a full minute licking, kissing, stroking or sucking that area to see just how excited they get and what really turns them on. Don't always choose the most obvious areas – this game is a brilliant opportunity to find some as yet undiscovered erogenous zones.

Blind Man's Buff

Remember the children's game Blind Man's Bluff? Well, this is the adult version, and definitely best when it's two players only. Ask your lover to strip, or gently help him or her to undress. Then put a blindfold on him or her and say that you're going to wrap him or her up. Using a combination of special bondage tape (that you can buy over the net at most sex toy shops) and standard cling film, wrap the tape around his or her wrists and ankles and then proceed to wrap the rest of his or her body (not the face, of course!) in the cling film, making it extra taut over the chest or breasts, bottom, thighs and genitals. It's visually stimulating for you, as seeing a body through a transparent casing can be very arousing. Then writhe all over your partner, so they can tantalisingly feel your flesh through the cling film but don't get the usual sensation of skin touching skin.

Strip Poker

This is a classic sex game that you were probably introduced to in college! However, it's even better played in a couples situation, especially if you factor in a few customised forfeits, insisting on the order of clothes removal, for example, or you can stroke and lick whichever part of the body becomes exposed, but stop the moment you see a sign of arousal like erect nipples or a moan of pleasure.

Let's look at the basic rules of poker and how you can get the maximum enjoyment out of a game of strip poker with your partner.

One of you is the dealer, and shuffles up a complete deck of cards. They deal five cards to you and five cards for them, all face down. Each of you then has the option to discard up to three cards and have them replaced with fresh cards from the top of the pack. Then you both reveal your hands and the person with the lowest hand has to take off an item of clothing before the game continues. The game continues in this fashion until one of you is entirely naked.

Straight flush

A straight flush is five cards in order, such as 7-8-9-10-J, all of the same suit. Aces can be high or low. An ace-high straight flush is called a Royal Flush and is the highest natural hand.

Four of a kind

Four cards of the same rank, e.g., four aces or four kings. If both your hands qualify, the hand with the highest rank four wins.

Full house

A full house is a three of a kind and a pair, such as K-K-K-2-2. When there are two full houses, the tie is broken by the higher-ranking three of a kind.

Flush

A hand in which all the cards are the same suit, such as 5-7-9-J-Q, all of diamonds. When there are two or more flushes, the flush containing the highest card wins.

Straight

Five cards in rank order, such as A-2-3-4-5, but not of the same suit. Aces can be high or low. When there are two straights, the highest straight wins. If two straights have the same value, the pot is split.

Three of a kind

Three cards of any rank, with the remaining cards not a pair. As with the full house, the highest-ranking three of a kind wins.

Two pairs

Two distinct pairs and a fifth card. The higher-ranking pair wins ties. If both hands have the same high pair, the second pair wins. If both hands have the same pairs, the high card (see below) wins.

Pair

One pair, with three other cards. The highest-ranking pair wins. High card breaks ties. When no player has even a pair, it comes down to whoever is holding the highest-ranking card. If there is a tie for the high card, the next high card determines the pot.

Roll The Dice

This involves a bit of artsy-crafty preparation, but getting ready is part of the fun. Buy two giant dice from a toy shop and then cover the six numbers of one die with labels of different, sexy body parts: genitals, nipples, tongue, neck, bottom and stomach. Then cover the six numbers of the other die with sex actions: suck, lick, nibble, kiss, caress and touch, for example. Take turns to throw the dice. You might get suck and nipples or lick and genitals.

Another exciting but challenging variation on this theme, which can work wonders for extra variety in your sex life, is to label one die with sexual acts – such as hand job, oral sex, making love, kissing, stroking and stripping – and the other one labelled with parts of the house – stairs, spare bedroom, bathroom, living room, dining room, etc.

Pleasure Hunt

Blindfold your partner and ask them to lie naked on the bed, face up or down as you choose. Let them relax as much as possible and then trace over their bare skin with a variety of objects, asking them whether they like it and to guess what you are stroking them with. Get a good selection of props ready for this before you start – ideas for props include a feather, a flower, a pearl necklace, a silk scarf, a leather paddle or crop, an ice cube, a piece of fake fur or your hair or another part of your body.

Honey Trap

This game requires a blindfold and a small amount of honey, chocolate sauce or golden syrup. And you'll need to be naked. Blindfold your partner, and then hide a drop of honey somewhere on your body. Without using his or her hands, and blindfolded, of course, your partner has to find that drop of honey with just their lips and tongue.

I Scream . . .

Buy half a dozen different ice-cream flavours and leave
them out of the freezer for 15 minutes before you play
this game. This game is going to get messy, so perhaps
it's best not done on your expensive Egyptian cotton
sheets! Now blindfold your partner while you dollop a
blob of different flavoured ice cream on various parts of
your body. He or she has to guess the flavour. When a
correct guess is made, it's your turn to be blindfolded
while you lick the ice cream off his or her body.

Peeping Tom

This game exploits your exhibitionist streak and your
partner's voyeuristic tendencies! Slowly take off your
clothes, as sensually as you can, while your partner views
your 'strip tease' from a hiding place, through a window
or behind an open door. He or she needs to keep very
quiet and still, as you 'don't know' that your lover is
watching you. When you've removed most or all of your
clothes, lie down on the bed or sofa and start to
masturbate.

Sexy Scrabble

You'll want to throw the ordinary rules of Scrabble out
the window for this game as getting the right spelling is
not the object of this game! No, the only rules are that

the words have to be sex-related, and the naughtier the better! Don't just stick to body parts descriptive words such as lick, nibble, caress and suck also work well. The winner gets to choose exactly which words on the board he or she gets to 'do' to you.

Sexy Treasure Chest

Keep a box full of sex memories. By saving items from great nights you've had together – ticket stubs or a programme from a concert or the receipt from a particularly memorable meal – you can look through these with your partner and remember what a great high you were on, and the really memorable sex you enjoyed together. These memories, in turn, can inspire you to find ways of repeating those evenings.

Or keep a list of shared desires and memories, which you can return to and revise from time to time, as your sex life gets more varied and adventurous. Share your current memories by asking each other questions and writing down the answers to keep in the 'chest', old shoe box or wherever you can keep these memories safe and accessible.

Divide your lists into four categories: *Locations*, *Times*, *Techniques* and *Playthings*. For example:

Location

- Best sex session in your bedroom . . .
- Best sex session elsewhere in your house . . .
- Best sex session away from your home . . .
- Most unusual place you've had sex . . .

Times

- Your first time together . . .
- A special occasion . . .
- Most fun together . . .
- Your most steamy session . . .

Techniques

- Best position ever . . .
- Most bizarre position . . .
- Most energetic position . . .
- Most intense orgasm . . .

Playthings

- Best sex toy . . .
- Best sex game . . .
- Best fantasy . . .
- Best role play . . .

Truth Or Bare

Most of us have played the traditional version of Truth

Or Dare – often saucy enough in itself – but this version is all about playing out your sexual fantasies. Use some of the suggestion cards from a board game or invent your own. Fun suggestions include getting your partner to perform a lap dance, do a striptease or ask them what they'd really like to do to you. Try to avoid questions about past lovers and exes – this is not a game designed to make anyone feel jealous, self-conscious or inadequate in any way.

Spin The Bottle

A more sophisticated (but only just!) version of Truth Or Bare, but you do have the perfect excuse to polish off a bottle of wine first. Along with your empty wine bottle, grab a large piece of plain paper and draw a circle, about twice the size of the bottle, marking it into six equal sections. Write a sex suggestion in each of the six sections that either of you can perform – give your partner a French kiss lasting a minute or more, perform a lap dance/striptease for your partner or blindfold your partner and ask him or her to find an erogenous zone by touch only.

Read With Lover

Buy an erotic novel or collections of short stories – there are some good ones in the Black Lace series and published by Agent Provocateur. Take it in turns to read a few pages to each other, using your most seductive voice. Close your eyes while your partner is reading to you and imagine what being in the story really feels like. This can be an incredibly exciting feeling – often more stimulating than watching visual erotica or porn itself.

So there we are – hopefully an entertaining romp through enough fantasies, role play, toys and games to keep you having fun for a little while. It's important to remember that the choice of sex game is entirely a personal one – what works for you might not work so well for your partner. It's about experimentation, being open-minded and having fun. Some will have you laughing out loud; others might have you writhing in ecstasy. As long as it's making you and your partner feel good about your sex lives, then go ahead and enjoy . . .

Useful Websites

Given that 'sex' is the most commonly typed word into Google, closely followed by 'porn', you may find some interesting diversions along the way if you're looking for more info on sex games, toys, fantasies or role play.

The major websites, selling everything from a simple blindfold to an upmarket sex toy, include almost every product I have talked about in this book – and much, much more – as well as offering wide-ranging tips and advice, user-friendly and often user-rated information on their products, as well as an ultra discreet and efficient mail order service.

www.sextoys.co.uk
www.lovehoney.co.uk
www.onjoy.co.uk

There are also a huge number of manufacturers' websites, selling a wide range of sex toys and games.

Some are a bit daunting and overwhelming, but I do recommend:

www.jejoue.com
www.ohmibod.com
www.lelo.com
www.funfactory.co.uk
www.jimmyjane.com
www.nookii.com
www.riskyorfrisky.com
www.bijouxindiscrets.com
www.creativeconceptions.co.uk
www.eroscillator.com

Acknowledgements

So, who to say thank you to when my latest book is written? Especially given the subject . . . So I'm going to keep it short and sweet.

Heartfelt thanks to my wonderful and closest friends who greeted the subject of this book with enthusiasm, curiosity, more than a few bottles of chilled white wine and a healthy 'Call that a job?!' attitude – Chris, Clare, Joanna, Jo, Carole, Tina, Monica, Sally, Pat, Sandra, Tara, Sarah and Rachel. And to Robert – whose frequent visits from New York meant he had to stay in a spare room stuffed to the rafters with sex toys. Tough luck, Rob . . .

Many thanks to my brilliant agent Liz and her team at Media Ambitions and my literary agent Amanda at Bonomi Associates and of course Julia, Jenny and Louise at Ebury, who did a brilliant job of editing, shaping up and promoting my ramblings.

My sanity (and the occasional undisciplined diversion) was often preserved by having a few rants on Twitter – so to those supportive virtual friends, some of whom I have had the pleasure of meeting face-to-face, thanks for your support, your humour and your retweets. For those who want to join in, you can find my meanderings on Twitter@TVpsychologist.

For those who never hesitate to provide fantastic advice, support, toys, games and props, I am indebted to Ruth Wilkinson at lovehoney.co.uk and Monique Carty at sextoys.co.uk. And huge thanks to Amy, Chris and the product development team at Philips, Dan at JeJoue, Nikki at Nookii, Melanie at Sexopoly, Jane at Creativeconceptions, Molly at Jimmyjane, Stephanie at Funfactory and Vicky at Lelo.

Finally, to my own, real-time, living, breathing, lovely man – thank you so much for being such a willing plaything.

Index

Index